THE DIABETIC WOMAN

Also by June Biermann and Barbara Toohey

THE DIABETIC'S BOOK: ALL YOUR QUESTIONS
ANSWERED
THE WOMAN'S HOLISTIC HEADACHE RELIEF BOOK
THE DIABETIC'S SPORTS & EXERCISE BOOK
THE DIABETES QUESTION & ANSWER BOOK
THE DIABETIC'S TOTAL HEALTH BOOK
THE PERIPATETIC DIABETIC

Under the name Margaret Bennett

BIKING FOR GROWNUPS
CROSS-COUNTRY SKIING FOR THE FUN OF IT
HOW TO SKI JUST A LITTLE BIT
DR. OWL'S PROBLEM
FROM BAEDEKER TO WORSE
ALICE IN WOMANLAND

Also by Lois Jovanovic, M.D.
(with Charles M. Peterson, M.D.)

THE DIABETES SELF-CARE METHOD
CONTEMPORARY ISSUES IN NUTRITION: DIABETES
MELLITUS
DIABETES IN PREGNANCY: TERATOLOGY, TOXICOLOGY,
AND TREATMENT
THE WOMAN'S ANSWER BOOK

THE
DIABETIC
WOMAN

Lois Jovanovic, M.D.
June Biermann
Barbara Toohey

JEREMY P. TARCHER, INC.
Los Angeles
Distributed by St. Martin's Press
New York

To Priscilla White,
who devoted her entire career as a physician
to the diabetic woman.

Library of Congress Cataloging in Publication Data

Jovanovic, Lois.
  The diabetic woman.

  —Bibliography
  Includes index.
  1. Diabetes—Popular works. 2. Women—Diseases.
I. Biermann, June. II. Toohey, Barbara. III. Title.
[DNLM: 1. Diabetes Mellitus—popular works. WK 850 J86w]
RC660.J64 1987   616.4'62   86-30092
ISBN 0-87477-411-X
ISBN 0-87477-410-1 (pbk.)

Jeremy P. Tarcher, Inc.
9110 Sunset Blvd.
Los Angeles, CA 90069

Design by Deborah Daly

Manufactured in the United States of America
10 9 8 7 6 5 4 3 2 1

First Edition

CONTENTS

Pregnancy. Husbands' Concerns. Effect on Children and Family. Economics of Pregnancy. Age at Pregnancy. Self-Care during Pregnancy. "Big Bad Baby" Syndrome. Cesarean Delivery. Number of Children. Adoption. Husband's Stress. Blood-Sugar Levels and Damage to Unborn Child. Ideal Blood Sugars during Pregnancy. Glycosylated Hemoglobin Test during Pregnancy. Pump during Pregnancy. Breast-Feeding.

Troisième Âge
Type II Risks. Blood-Sugar-Lowering Pills. Insulin as Type II Treatment. Type I Insulin Reactions. Menopause. Hormone Replacement. Weight Gain After Menopause. Psychological Problems. Heart Disease.

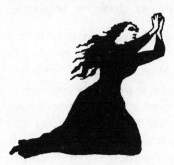

Please...
READ THE
INTRODUCTIONS

As former librarians and avid readers ourselves, we know how people read a book. Almost everyone skips the material up front—the dedications, forewords, prefaces, and introductions. They figure this is just a lot of boring stuff, such as acknowledgments to everyone who has happened to cross the author's path since she or he first picked up a pen or laid fingers to a typewriter or word processor, or else it's a lot of background information that's too tedious to be worked into the body of the book. People also tend to skim and dip into the body of a book —particularly a nonfiction book—looking for the things that interest them most or perhaps for the so-called "good parts" (note: the material on sex can be found in chapter 2!).

With this book we urge you to break the normal reading pattern and read the introductions. They're not long and won't take much time, but we feel they will give you an understanding of why this book was written and how we found what questions needed answering. Most important, you'll learn something about Lois Jovanovic and about why she is probably the most qualified person on earth to answer a diabetic woman's questions.

Then, because we feel *everything* in the book is important for you to read—even those sections that at first glance may seem somewhat irrelevant to your diabetes and your life—we hope you'll follow the reading advice from *Alice in Wonderland.* "Begin at the beginning, and go on until you come to the end: then stop."

After that you can skim and dip and reread the sections most important to you until diabetes control becomes second nature to you. Then, once and for all, you will have changed your emphasis from

DIABETIC woman
to
diabetic **WOMAN**

and you'll be ready to plunge into the whole exciting spectrum of experiences that life has to offer you.

June Biermann
Barbara Toohey
Van Nuys,
California

CHERCHEZ LA FEMME

by June Biermann and Barbara Toohey

Because we've written four books on diabetes, people often write to us suggesting other books that are needed and that they wish we would write. The one book that has been suggested over and over is a book on the woman diabetic, on how to handle all the unique problems of being a diabetic along with all the unique problems of being a woman.

We realized the need but frankly didn't feel capable of the task. For all our previous books we used June as the guinea pig, telling about her diagnosis and coming to terms with diabetes in *The Peripatetic Diabetic,* answering all the basic questions about diabetes and diabetes therapy in *The Diabetic's Book,* reporting her experiences and those of more than 100 other sports-minded, active diabetics in *The Diabetic's Sports and Exercise Book,* and presenting an approach concentrating on health rather than illness in *The Diabetic's Total Health Book.*

We felt confident and capable in those areas, but June just didn't have the total experience necessary for us to counsel all women with diabetes. Since her diabetes was diagnosed at age forty-five, she couldn't describe what it was like to go through the upheavals of puberty while trying to keep diabetes in control, nor could she describe what it was like to be a young wife juggling diabetes along with all her other growing responsibilities. June had no children—and if she had, she would have had them before becoming diabetic and thus could not make any personal contributions on that most crucial issue of how a diabetic woman has a successful pregnancy. She couldn't even give firsthand reports about going through menopause, because she'd had a hysterectomy a year before her diabetes was discovered. (We've often thought that the hysterectomy might have been the stress that pulled the trigger on her diabetes-loaded genetic gun.)

No, we definitely didn't have the experiential wherewithal needed for a book on the diabetic woman. We often discussed the issue. What we really had to have, we finally decided, was a collaborator. That ideal collaborator would be a diabetic woman endocrinologist specializing in diabetes. She would need to be up-to-date on the latest developments in the field, but she shouldn't be so fresh from her residency that she wouldn't have the in-depth background of having worked with a large number of patients. We wanted her to be married, and we wanted her to have children—and to have given birth to them when she was a diabetic. We wanted her to be a warm and compassionate person who would have empathy for every problem—no matter how minor it might seem—that a diabetic woman might have. We wanted her to be a clear thinker and a graceful writer with a practical turn of mind. We wanted her to be someone oriented toward working with people, not strictly a researcher who looked at everything in terms of studies done with rats. And we wanted her to have a sense of humor—we knew we could never work with someone who didn't have that!

Even we had to laugh at our outrageous demands. How could we ever expect to find such a paragon? Eternal optimists that we are, though, we put a notice in our Sugarfree Center *Health-O-Gram* saying that we were trying to find the name of a diabetic woman diabetologist. We didn't go into all the other requirements we had. Even so, we heard nothing; apparently, not even a shadow of the person we needed existed. We pushed the project to the back of our minds.

Nevertheless, our women readers and clients at the Sugarfree Center kept asking questions, so we kept muttering to friends in the diabetes health professions that we sure wished we could find a diabetic woman physician specializing in diabetes. One day our mutterings and our prayers were answered. Our Nordisk Insulin representative, Tom Avery, asked, "Isn't Lois Jovanovic a diabetic woman?" and then, answering his own question, he said, "Yes, I'm sure she is."

Our first lead! Although Dr. Jovanovic was on the East Coast and we were on the West, her name was familiar to us. We thought we remembered that she worked with the eminent diabetologist Dr. Charles Peterson at Rockefeller University. This was confirmed when we received a copy of a new book, *The Diabetes Self-Care Method,* which doctors Peterson and Jovanovic had written together. We were extremely impressed by the book and excited by the fact that Dr. Jovanovic was a good writer and collaborator. Although nowhere in the book was it mentioned that one of the authors actually was a diabetic woman, we were particularly attracted by one illustration, a close-up of four pristine-looking fingertips. The caption was: "These are the tips of the fingers of a diabetic person who for the past eight years has monitored her own blood glucose." We suspected whose fingertips they were.

All these seemed like sufficiently good omens for us

to begin our tentative "collaboration dances" with Dr. Jovanovic. We asked our editor to get in touch and see if she might be interested in working with us, because we didn't want her to feel put on the spot, as she would be if we asked her directly. The answer was that Dr. Jovanovic was not only very enthusiastic about the idea of the collaboration but, according to our editor, she had also said that she had enjoyed our books. That took care of the sense of humor problem. No physician without one would have the slightest taste for our writing.

As we got closer to the collaboration, we received a biographical sketch that revealed Dr. Jovanovic's credentials to be even beyond our original outrageous demands: B.S. in Biology from Columbia University; M.D. from Albert Einstein College of Medicine; intern and resident in internal medicine at New York Hospital; research fellow in endocrinology and metabolism at Cornell University Medical College, and later instructor and then associate professor in obstetrics/gynecology at that same institution; guest investigator at Rockefeller University; and soon, as convenience would have it, she was moving West to be senior scientist at the Sansum Medical Research Foundation in Santa Barbara—near us. She'd also written enough professional articles on diabetes to choke a library. We later found out that, in addition to all of the above, as a physician Dr. Jovanovic had been involved with more than 130 diabetic pregnancies (half of which resulted in babies named Lois!). And *two* of the pregnancies she had been involved with were her own. Bingo.

And so it happened that despite the fact that we'd never met Dr. Jovanovic face-to-face, we agreed to collaborate on *The Diabetic Woman.* Our first meeting with Lois—as we had come to think of her—took place in New York at the American Diabetes Association 33rd Postgraduate Course where she was a featured speaker.

When we first saw Lois we realized that her age was exactly as we had ordered. She was youthful—probably in her early thirties—and, except for the braid, she looked like the description of her written by Gennell Subak-Sharpe in the book *Living With Diabetes:* "Dr. Jovanovic arrives, looking more like a pert schoolgirl than a doctor, with her long dark hair worn in a single braid and a brightly colored scarf tied around her waist." And she was obviously experienced. We were awed by her presentation at the meeting, deciding that she must have put in untold hours of preparation to make her talk—as well as her responses to questions from the audience—smooth, lucid, and fraught with information. Here was a woman who had it all in her head and right at her fingertips, to mix metaphors.

Although we had confidence at this point that Lois was right for the book, it wasn't until a few weeks later that for us the whipped cream was put on the collaborative sundae.

We had written to ask Lois some specific questions. When she called she apologized for not getting in touch sooner, explaining that she'd had to go to the office to use the phone because her new puppy had chewed through the telephone cord. "What kind of dog do you have?" asked Barbara (with visions frolicking in her head of something appropriately exotic for a noted endocrinologist: a Lhasa apso, maybe, or a komondor).

"Oh, I don't know what she is," Lois replied. "I just went to the pound and took the first puppy who licked my face."

At that moment we knew for sure that we'd found our woman—and yours.

TRUE CONFESSIONS

by Lois Jovanovic, M.D.

My father had Type I diabetes. By the time he had children, he was already riddled with problems. I remember his morning ritual of testing his urine—with a tablet, which I now know was Clinitest. The test tube became very hot, and the contents then turned an ugly brown or orange. Now I realize that he never, never was in good control. He took his insulin with a glass syringe, which mother boiled. Every afternoon he had an insulin reaction (insulin shock caused by extremely low blood sugar), and if we didn't rush home from school to give him dinner, he was in diabetic coma.

From my earliest memories, daddy was bedridden and blind. At the time of his death, I was twelve; he was fifty, with twenty years of diabetes. I promised at his graveside that I would devote my life to curing diabetes.

At almost the exact age at which my father got his diabetes, I developed mine. I had completed medical school and medical residency and was in the middle of my endocrine/metabolism fellowship when it happened to me.

I completely denied the symptoms. I attributed my weight loss, irritability, and insomnia (which was caused by my constant need to urinate during the night) to the stress of my career.

Then, during the middle of an experiment, I donated my blood as a normal control. When it came back sky-high—more than three times the normal range—I thought the assay was wrong. When my blood was used to calibrate the biostator (a kind of giant mechanical pancreas used in hospitals), I did not think that the 400 blood sugar might be mine but instead screamed at the technician that she was not calibrating the machine correctly.

After three months of deteriorating health, I was forced by a dear friend and colleague to accept the truth. I refused, however, to admit that I needed insulin. I was sure that I could manage my "mild diabetes" with diet (in essence, starvation), exercise, and, if necessary, oral agents. In less than a week I was in ketoacidotic coma, that advanced state of out-of-control diabetes that can lead to death if insulin is not given.

Denial was certainly the major component in the onset of my diabetes. The next stages were all in accordance with the classic stages described in Elisabeth Kübler-Ross's book *On Death and Dying*. I went through the phases of anger and depression and finally arrived at recovery and acceptance. This process took me a year. Now I know that a year of grief is normal when a chronic disease is diagnosed.

I didn't really change my career plans, but I refused to "come out of the closet." The truth was difficult to admit publicly. I thought my credibility as a physician and a scientist would be harmed. I only revealed my diabetes five years ago, when I went on a big, big insulin pump. Then I *couldn't* deny my "affliction"!

Surprisingly, I found out that my diabetes actually

enhanced my credibility. Not only were physicians more respectful but in addition patients became more willing to follow my advice, since they knew I was following it myself.

Perhaps my acceptance took too long—but then again, I saw my father crippled by the disease, and thus it was terrifying to me. And it did serve to make me understanding of denial in other diabetic people and to allow me to be better able to help them work through theirs.

I haven't cured diabetes, nor has anyone else—yet. I have all faith, though, that someone will find a cure in the not-too-distant future. In the meantime, your goal should be to stay healthy and to keep your blood sugar normal so that you'll be ready to enjoy the benefits of that cure. Your other goal should be to lead a wonderful life. What, after all, is the good of being a perfect diabetic woman if it means sacrificing all the joys of human existence?

I know from my own personal experience, as June knows from hers, that these two goals—good control and a wonderful life—are not incompatible. They *can* be achieved. My goal in this book is to help you achieve them.

CHAPTER
1

WHAT EVERY DIABETIC WOMAN SHOULD KNOW

We don't think of this book as being directed specifically to the woman who knows nothing or next to nothing about diabetes. (See Recommended Reading in Appendix A for a list of good, easy-to-read basic books for the beginning diabetic woman.) Still, we realize that some newly diagnosed women are very likely to come across this book and read it before reading any other. Therefore, we want to start off with a brief rundown of the what's, who's, and why's of diabetes. This may also be good information for women who have had diabetes for quite a while but who may have some ideas that are out of date or even flat-out wrong. As the rustic philosopher Josh Billings put it, "It iz better tew know nothing than tew know what ain't so."

After a brief review of the basics, we'll go on to a discussion of the questions that concern every woman with diabetes, no matter what age she may be or what kind of life she may be leading: active or passive; career outside the home, inside the home, or both; married, single, or divorced; mother or not.

Dr. Jovanovic, please lead off by telling us just what this thing called diabetes is.

Dr. Jovanovic: Diabetes mellitus means "flowing of honey." It refers to the copious amount of urine produced when the blood glucose (level of sugar in the bloodstream) is high. Diabetes mellitus is, therefore, the name given to a disease characterized by a high blood-sugar level.

June and Barbara: Just how high is high enough for a person to be categorized as diabetic?

Dr. Jovanovic: The diagnosis of diabetes is usually based on a glucose-tolerance test. This test consists of 75 grams of sugar given as a drink, with blood tests drawn before the drink and one, two, and three hours after it.

The arbitrary cutoff established by the National Diabetes Data Group in 1979 stated that diabetes mellitus is defined as a fasting plasma glucose above 140 milligrams per deciliter (mg/dl) and/or any plasma glucose that is above 200 mg/dl after two or three hours have elapsed.

With these levels as the cutoffs, anyone whose blood-sugar levels are higher receives the label of "diabetic." How the blood sugars became high is another matter.

If the blood sugar rose because the person's pancreas failed to secrete enough insulin, then the person is classified as a Type I diabetic person. If the person has a high blood sugar because she or he cannot get rid of the sugar once it's ingested—in other words, has a clearance problem—then the person has Type II diabetes.

Two other forms of diabetes are possible. Gestational diabetes is the diabetes that has its onset during pregnancy and goes away after pregnancy. Secondary diabetes is that diabetes resulting from another disease.

Once the other disease is cured, then the diabetes goes away. Classic examples of secondary diabetes include Cushing's disease (a disease characterized by too much cortisol, a hormone made in the adrenal gland), acromegaly (giantism), and pheochromocytoma (a vascular tumor of the adrenal medulla).

It's important that not only the diagnosis of diabetes be made but also the correct classification in order to help guide the best therapy to normalize the high glucose levels. Type I diabetic persons require insulin therapy; Type II diabetic persons may do well on diet, exercise, and/or oral agents (blood-sugar-lowering pills).

June and Barbara: Are the symptoms of Type I and Type II diabetes different?

Dr. Jovanovic: Yes. When a person develops Type I diabetes, the effects of hyperglycemia (high blood sugar) are manifest immediately: great thirst and urination, constant hunger, massive weight loss, and irritability. If the diabetes isn't treated with immediate insulin therapy, the irritability will turn to disorientation, coma, and eventual death.

Type II diabetes creeps up gradually, and symptoms are therefore tolerated. A person may not be bothered by the high blood sugars until these high blood-glucose levels cause other problems, like vaginitis or foot infections. These symptoms confirm the diagnosis but are not necessary to it.

June and Barbara: June's symptoms were that subtle kind. She, who was normally healthy to a fault, kept getting sore throats and colds that lingered and lingered. Incidentally, because her symptoms were gradual and because she was forty-five when her diabetes was diagnosed, we think of her as a Type II. And yet she did have to go on insulin. We have a theory, based strictly on observation, that the Type IIs who are thin generally have to go on insulin, while the overweight ones can often control their diabetes through diet, exercise, and sometimes pills after losing their excess weight. We've heard that the French categorize diabetics as *"maigres"* (thins) and *"gras"* (fats) rather than as Type I and Type II. Their belief is that the *maigres* usually have to go on insulin and that the *gras* usually don't. Do you agree with this?

Dr. Jovanovic: Yes, I agree, although some Type IIs are really Type Is who are on their way to complete pancreatic "poopout" and thus need insulin all along. Other thin Type IIs *are* really thin Type IIs, and with rigorous exercise, a low-carbohydrate diet, and the oral hypoglycemic agents, they can squeak by without insulin. But insulin is the best treatment for the majority of thin Type IIs.

Fat Type IIs have plenty of insulin coming from their pancreases. Their problem is that they cannot clear the sugar after it is eaten. The treatment of choice for them is to restrict their amount of food so that the sugar does not build up in the bloodstream.

June and Barbara: A woman who got "instant diabetes" from having 85 percent of her pancreas removed complained to us that her surgeon and family doctor disagree on the long-term outlook, and she can find no information on this form of diabetes. Could you, as they say, compare and contrast (as they like to put it on college essay examinations) surgically induced diabetes with the standard variety?

Dr. Jovanovic: Sometimes surgical removal of the pancreas (pancreatectomy) is necessary in the case of pancreatic carcinoma, insulinomas, and certain forms of pancreatitis (infectious), specifically, idiopathic (of unknown cause) and/or alcoholic pancreatitis. In these cases, when the pancreas is removed all of the pancreatic functions are removed, not just the insulin-producing cells. The pancreas also makes digestive enzymes. When these are removed, the result is a malabsorption syndrome. This syndrome includes protein and fat wasting, plus deficiencies of vitamins A, D, E, and K because these vitamins are absorbed with fat in the gut. In addition, glucagon, the hormone that raises blood sugar, which is produced by the alpha cells in the pancreas, is missing. Thus, this diabetes is difficult to manage for many reasons.

The insulin requirement is usually one-half to two-thirds less for a person whose pancreas has been removed than for a Type I diabetic person, since without glucagon there is not the usual buffer against insulin action. These patients can go into DKA (diabetic ketoacidosis), despite the old teaching that DKA is associated with elevated glucagon levels. These people prove that DKA is the result of absolute insulin lack.

People whose pancreases have been surgically removed are exquisitely brittle (unstable). They can go very low with a low dose of insulin, because the food they eat does not get into their bloodstream due to the lack of digestive enzymes.

June and Barbara: Sometimes when people are first diagnosed as having diabetes they race to a dictionary or encyclopedia and by mistake read about diabetes insipidus, which has nothing to do with their condition. To alleviate this confusion could you explain what that other disease, diabetes insipidus, is?

Dr. Jovanovic: Diabetes insipidus is also a disease characterized by massive urination. The cause of this urination, however, is a lack of a hormone called vasopressin or antidiuretic hormone. The posterior pituitary gland makes this hormone, and if a tumor destroys the posterior pituitary, water is spontaneously lost from the kidneys.

June and Barbara: We've always understood that more women than men have diabetes, but at the ADA (American Diabetes Association) Conference where we heard you speak, we also heard a talk at which it was pointed out that in Europe men are now in the majority.

Dr. Jovanovic: For Type I diabetics, it's usually fifty-fifty, but at times it changes to forty-sixty or sixty-forty. It's like the gender swings in baby booms.

For Type II it's more likely to be 65 to 70 percent women and 30 to 35 percent men.

June and Barbara: Why us?

Dr. Jovanovic: Women have more body fat than men, even in the normal weight range (25 to 30 percent in women versus 18 to 25 percent in men). Increased body fat increases your chances for diabetes when the heredity is there. In the abnormal ranges, women tend to be more obese than men. They also tend to gain weight during pregnancy, and this weight is often not entirely shed afterward.

There is also the factor that Type II diabetes is inherited more from the mother's side than from the father's side.

June and Barbara: One diabetic sociologist of our acquaintance maintains that women have more diabetes than men because of the stresses of being pulled in every direction, trying to fill every role that society seems to require of them: housekeeper, gourmet cook, lover and companion to her husband, mother, career woman, etc. She says that no matter what a woman is doing at a given moment, she feels guilty because she's not doing something else. Do you think those stresses could be a factor in bringing out diabetes?

Dr. Jovanovic: Of course, if you try to be a superwoman, that's going to create stress, and stress does bring out and exacerbate diabetes. I've heard of a new organization in San Francisco called "Superwomen Anonymous," founded by Carol Orsborn, author of *Enough Is Enough: Exploding the Myth of Having It All.* This organization is geared toward helping women who are caught up in trying to have it all. Maybe joining that would be a help for stressed-out diabetic women. But stress isn't exclusive to the female sex. Some of my male patients double their insulin requirement during the week of April 15. It's more a matter of the individual and her or his ability to cope with the stresses that assail everyone in modern society.

June and Barbara: Yes, coping is the key. You know, way back in 1980 we wrote an entire book, *The Diabetic's Total Health Book*, focusing on the role of stress in diabetes. Because of June's personal experience and stories we heard from other diabetics we saw the devastating effects of the stressors of contemporary life on chronic health problems such as diabetes. We presented in that book a smorgasbord of relaxation therapies, beginning with the biofeedback technique that you tried in your study and continuing with progressive relaxation, autogenic training, meditation, guided imagery, and such unorthodox methods as laughter and hug therapy. All of these techniques work if you practice them regularly. You just have to discover which ones work best for you and then— here's the crucial factor—take or make time to do them.

Recently, June has been getting excellent control of her condition by switching from needle to jet injection of insulin. This has produced a predictable result from her normal dosage and has enabled her to keep 90 percent or more of her blood-sugar readings at a normal level. But about 10 percent—and on some days even more—of her blood sugars still remain above normal levels. Why? It's all because of unusual pressures on those days. Now she laughs and says, "I'm no longer testing my blood sugar. I'm testing my stress level." And, believe us, she has resumed her meditation sessions, which she had been blithely skipping in order to "get more done."

Dr. Jovanovic: We advised the patients in our study to use biofeedback relaxation twice a day and whenever a difficult situation arose in their lives. We did learn one exception to the effectiveness of stress reduction therapies. None of our patients could control their blood-sugar levels in times of catastrophic events. We learned that when something really traumatic happens—death of a loved one, car accident, robbery, fire, school failure, etc.—it is normal to forget diabetes self-care and relaxation techniques. The crisis takes precedence, making it impossible to think of anything but the disaster itself. Therefore, it is best to cope with the disaster and avoid feeling guilty about transient loss of diabetes control. Then, when the crisis has passed, diabetes control can take center stage once more.

June and Barbara: A number of people would put you in the superwoman category, since you are a physician, wife, and mother, along with your many other roles. Do you find that when you're under heavy stress, your blood sugars tend to go up and/or you need to increase your insulin?

Dr. Jovanovic: Yes, I do wax and wane when stress appears, but my eating habits tend to change when I am under stress, so it's hard to figure out entirely. I must say that my insulin requirement has dropped 10 percent now that I'm a "laid back" Californian instead of a high-powered New Yorker. This decreased insulin requirement is even more amazing because I have also gained weight. I guess stress did contribute a bit to my overall control.

I participated in a study of biofeedback relaxation [published in *Diabetes Care,* November-December 1985] in which relaxation exercises did decrease the insulin requirement and improve the instability of glucose levels up to 20 percent in selected patients.

Incidentally, many diabetics don't realize that diabetes is itself a great stress factor. You have to worry about high and low blood sugars and you have to remember to have food along wherever you go, as well as your insulin and testing materials. Diabetes is always there in the back of your mind, and that builds up the stress level.

June and Barbara: In a letter we received, a woman pointed out that there are both advantages and disadvantages to being a diabetic woman rather than a diabetic man. Her theory was that women have an advantage because they generally understand food better and also that they can make a better psychological adjustment to the disease because they don't have to present a tough macho image, which might make men ashamed to wear a pump or do something else that would help their control. On the other hand, she felt that women had a disadvantage in that it's usually hard for them to put themselves first, and as a result their diabetes is generally more unstable. Do you agree with her "good news, bad news" theory?

Dr. Jovanovic: Not entirely. I can't really think of why it might be an advantage to be a diabetic woman rather than a diabetic man. Women don't necessarily understand food. They know taste, quality, texture, color, freshness, and so forth. The nutrient value of food is not the main topic in Julia Child's gourmet cooking class. Both men and women take health class in junior high school, and it's as easy for a man to memorize food values as a woman. A man may not be in charge of the food he eats, but why should a man be in poor diabetic control because his wife seasons with sugar or honey? He could investigate the problem and solve it as well as a woman.

Now that the pumps are small enough to be easily hidden in a pocket, the issue of publicly wearing your diabetes is no longer a valid issue, macho feelings or not.

It's true, however, that the menstrual cycle changes the insulin requirement. The insulin therefore needs adjusting once a month for women, whereas men are pretty stable except during times of business stress, such as tax time, when the blood-glucose level can increase by two or three times. Also, pregnancy is a lot more complicated for a woman with diabetes than a man with diabetes!

I must admit, too, that it's often difficult for a woman to put herself first, since she's so accustomed to taking care of everyone else in the family.

June and Barbara: That's certainly true. We've noticed that it's often hard for a woman to take the time out to care for herself when she has a cold, let alone when she has something as time-consuming and inexorable as diabetes. We always maintain that you must take care of yourself or you won't be able to do anything for others.

If you aren't willing to make the effort to control your diabetes for yourself, how about doing it for those you love? In that way you can free them from worrying about your diabetes and allow them to live up to their fullest potential. The following note, which came attached to an announcement of the writer's graduation from law school, shows how very important your control can be to others. Although it's from a woman writing about her diabetic husband, it holds true for either sex.

> Dear June and Barbara:
>   We purchased a meter in December. Since then my husband's diabetes has been controlled. It certainly took a load of worry off my mind during my last year in law school. In that light I wanted to share my graduation with you. Thanks for all your help!

One young woman confessed to us that her husband had told her that she used to be disagreeable about half the time—"a real bitch" was how he put it. But since she had started controlling her blood sugar "she's become a wonderful human being and a joy to be around."

And while you're controlling your blood sugar for the benefit of others, you should start investigating why you don't control it for yourself. Don't you consider yourself important? Aren't you worth the effort? Don't you love yourself enough?

To return from psychology to physiology, one woman wrote to ask if more women than men are affected by diabetic neuropathy. The reason she asked was that many Type II diabetic women in her diabetes group developed neuropathy but none of the men did (although, she pointed out, men rarely attended the meetings).

Dr. Jovanovic: Type II diabetes is more common among women than men, so naturally more of them would develop neuropathy. But if the question is asked about Type I diabetics, men get neuropathy just as frequently as women.

June and Barbara: We think this is a rather minor controversy, but some otherwise rational people get quite shrill about it. Do you have any strong opinion, based on either your own feelings or those reported to you by your patients, about whether a person should say "I am a diabetic" or "I have diabetes"? June doesn't care one way or the other, but she usually says the former. Exponents of the "I have diabetes" school maintain that their diabetes is only a secondary consideration and feel that if they say, "I am a diabetic," it intrudes on the dignity of their personhood.

Dr. Jovanovic: Funny, I think the only people who are fussy about this are nondiabetics. I always say that it doesn't matter if I am a person with syphilis or if I am a syphilitic—I still have the same disease. Actually, it is incorrect to use the word *diabetic* as a noun, and the American Diabetes Association will not allow its use in this way. In the final analysis, I'm not particularly happy with any label.

June and Barbara: Enough of these nomenclatural shenanigans. Whether you call yourself a woman diabetic or a diabetic woman, what is the best type of doctor to see? An internist? A gynecologist? A diabetologist? An endocrinologist?

Dr. Jovanovic: Ideally, every diabetic woman should have the luxury of three doctors—a diabetologist, an internist, and a gynecologist—and one dentist.

However, depending on what area of the country she lives in and on her finances, a diabetic woman may be able to choose only one doctor. A well-trained internist should be able to adjust insulin or oral hypoglycemic agents, do Pap smears, and treat other ailments, too. But an internist often does not have adequate time, teaching materials, or support staff for intensive diabetes management. Thus, if a diabetic woman wants an intensified management program, she may be disappointed with the minimal interaction she may get related to diabetes issues.

June and Barbara: Incidentally, many people, ourselves included, are confused by the terms used for physicians specializing in diabetes. Many are called endocrinologists and others diabetologists. Are they the same?

Dr. Jovanovic: They *can* be the same, but they aren't always. Let me explain: an endocrinologist is board certified in that specialty by the American College of Physicians; a diabetologist is any physician who specializes in the treatment of diabetes and who mainly treats diabetics. An internist or general practitioner could be a diabetologist, as could an endocrinologist who specializes in diabetes.

June and Barbara: Going to the doctor seems to be stressful for everyone. Women (and men) who come into the Sugarfree Center like to tell us war stories about their doctors. Some of the doctors are portrayed as saints, but to be honest, a good percentage of the time he or she is made to sound like an avaricious devil who gives virtually no attention to the patient's problems. And we see the other side, too—patients who seem to feel that the doctor has an obligation to them, to the exclusion of all other patients, to give them infinite time for even the most infinitesimal complaints and to then charge only a token amount for their services.

It reminds us of when we were librarians in the Los Angeles Community College District. One of our colleagues wryly remarked, "The professors think they should be paid for staying at home, and the district thinks they should work for nothing." The answer has to lie somewhere in between. So must it lie somewhere in between for patients and doctors.

As a physician and a diabetic woman, you can see both sides of the picture. Could you give us an idea of what a diabetic patient has a legitimate right to expect from a doctor's visit?

Dr. Jovanovic: It also has something to do with being a woman as well as a diabetic. Women of necessity visit physicians more than men do. We're locked into a compulsory visit to the gynecologist for a Pap smear, and when we have babies numerous doctor visits are necessary.

Let's examine the case of a doctor's visit for a Pap smear. Although the purpose of this visit is to have a simple test, somehow we feel cheated if the doctor doesn't take time to talk to us and show concern. Thus, our expectations of what we think the purpose of this visit is are clearly different from what the doctor thinks the purpose of this visit is.

On top of a background of preconceived expectations, a diabetic woman visits a diabetes specialist. I shall now take the point of view of a physician and describe what I think should happen in the doctor's office, and then I'll describe my response as a diabetic woman who is given this care.

At the initial visit the doctor should take a complete history, including the following points:

Age
Duration of diabetes
Medications
Insulin history (A review of types of insulin and number of injections along with dosages and needs, especially if the times of the doses have significantly changed)
Number of episodes of ketoacidosis and need for hospitalizations

Number of severe hypoglycemia episodes and review of the most recent history of even minor hypoglycemia

Assessment of control—type of glucose monitoring done (urine or blood) and typical patterns over the years

History of complications of diabetes, specifically those related to the eyes, kidneys, feet, and nerves

Menstrual history—onset, frequency, character, and duration

Pregnancy-related history

Family history, not only of diabetes but also of heart disease, hypertension, and seizure disorders

Other coexisting illnesses

Previous surgery

History of allergies

History of severe infections: ear, pneumonia, urine, and/or kidney

Then the doctor should ask the patient the reason for the visit. Is it just a checkup? Does the patient want a change in insulin dosage? Is the patient seeking better control? Does the patient have a complication of diabetes that she is worried about? Based on the chief reason for the visit, the doctor will then direct more questions toward trying to come to an answer to the problems. The total time to take the history should be about fifteen to twenty minutes.

The initial visit should also include a complete physical examination, but one that's directed to diabetes-related problems:

Height, weight, blood pressure, pulse

Eyes: the back of the eye will be examined

Nose, ears, mouth, tongue, teeth, and skin

Neck: emphasis on thyroid and lymph glands

Chest: the doctor will listen with the stethoscope to both lungs and heart.

Abdomen: the doctor will check here for liver, spleen, and enlarged uterus and will listen with the stethoscope for bowel sounds and abnormal blood-vessel noises.

Groin area: pulses and lymph glands

Pelvic and rectal: the diabetes doctor will usually not do a pelvic or rectal examination but rather will confirm with the patient that she does have a gynecologist.

Legs and feet: these will be examined for pulses, muscle strength, and nerve function, including ankle and knee jerks and sensation and position sense.

The total time for the complete physical examination should be around fifteen to twenty minutes.

Based on the history and the physical, the doctor will formulate a problem list and a plan of attack. The patient will be asked to get dressed and then meet the doctor in the consultation room to learn about her problems and the possible solutions to them.

Let's assume that the patient came to the diabetes specialist for improvement of blood-sugar control and that she was well, with no complications of diabetes. The doctor would then first reinforce good preventive-care habits, including such basics as an eye-doctor appointment at least once a year, care with cutting toenails, etc.

The doctor would then set up a series of follow-up appointments to see that any suggested change in insulin dose meets the needs of the patient and to discuss the results of laboratory tests ordered. The essential laboratory tests include glycosylated hemoglobin (see related question later in this chapter), thyroid-function tests, kidney tests, blood count, and blood-chemistry tests.

Like the history and the physical, this discussion

period should last from fifteen to twenty minutes. Note that the doctor can by no means prescribe a "better" dose of insulin in this session. Instead, a stepwise plan should be created that includes education on diet, exercise, home blood-glucose monitoring, charting, sick-day procedures, and the like. Most of the educational interaction will be between the patient and the nurse and/or dietitian. Subsequent visits to the nurse and dietitian will probably be made when the doctor may not be available. Phone contact will likely be through the office nurse and may not be directly to the physician.

Once a patient's new diabetes program is under way (establishing a new program may take several closely spaced visits), a repeat visit should occur three to four times a year for checkup and laboratory blood tests. Each of these visits will be around twenty to thirty minutes long.

Now, how do I as a patient respond to the treatment described above? It depends on my expectations. If I thought the doctor was going to be my only health-care professional, I might resent the nurse and/or dietitian, although these people usually are better teachers than a busy doctor. Perhaps I came in for one visit to have my blood sugars fixed and found that my doctor couldn't give me a magic dose of insulin in one visit but insisted that I come back several times to visit his nurse, keep tedious records of my own blood tests, and stick to a rigid diet. On top of all the work that I was assigned, I was billed for each and every visit, even if I did not see the doctor. Never mind that my blood-sugar level improved.

Rather than experience a series of disappointments, it would be better to begin the first visit by telling the doctor what you expect and then having the doctor tell you what will happen. Then, with agreement, you and the doctor can problem solve together.

June and Barbara: That covers the physiological aspects of a diabetic woman's visit to the doctor. Now, how about the emotional aspects? Could you imagine for us that you're in the office with a Type I diabetic woman who is either newly diagnosed or who has had diabetes for a year or less?

Dr. Jovanovic: It's not hard for me to imagine this scene, since I've often had the occasion to consult with patients within a year of their diagnosis. Unfortunately, I find that as a whole the health-professional community hasn't met the needs of a woman who is given the diagnosis of a chronic disease at a young age.

Just as there are five stages of grieving when a person loses a loved one, there are five stages of grieving when a person is confronted with the diagnosis of diabetes. Stage one is disbelief and denial. Much of this stage is spent arguing with the Almighty and negotiating a reprieve. Stage two is anger. Why me? Stage three is depression and withdrawal. Stage four is recovery, and stage five is acceptance. It usually takes a year to complete the entire process of grief.

I usually meet the women during their depression. They are even more depressed because their previous doctor usually hasn't allowed such indulgence in "self-pity." They get reprimands and rejection from their doctors instead of the support they so desperately need. This intensifies their depression.

Nothing seems to help more than my telling these women that a year for the entire grief process is the norm and that some people take longer. This rids them of false feelings of guilt or of the conviction that their behavior is weak or aberrant.

I've also often heard from patients that they have been told their diabetes is too mild for an intensive program of care. As a result, they're given no education about the rationale for controlling blood sugar or about how it is to be achieved. They're not even asked if they prefer an intensive program.

The last, and probably the worst, problem is the fear these women have about asking simple questions that emerge from the soul. Will I be impotent? Lose my legs? Be blind and die on a kidney machine? These are very real fears for a woman who has read about diabetes in the women's magazines before she knew that one day she would develop the disease. Merely telling patients that most complications of diabetes do not happen for five to ten years after the diagnosis is a relief to most newly diagnosed persons. Then a teachable moment is reached in which I can make a plug for good glucose control to reinforce that the woman is keeper of her own fate and that she does not have to be a victim of her own disease.

It would be unfair to the woman, however, if I didn't admit to her that there are a few problems that do happen immediately. High blood sugar increases anxiety and irritability and requires greater coping skills. I can assure her, though, that the unstable personality she's now experiencing can be helped by stabilizing her blood-sugar levels. Better blood sugar can also help any uncomfortable vaginitis she may be experiencing. It's worth it for me to adjust a patient's therapy to alleviate these two problems alone, even if it means more than one injection a day of insulin.

June and Barbara: We've noticed that diabetic women tend to blame every physical problem they have—from dandruff to hangnails—on their diabetes. Are there certain conditions in which a woman is justified in accusing her diabetes?

Dr. Jovanovic: Let's not say diabetes, but *out-of-control* diabetes. There's a vast difference between the two. Well-controlled diabetes is usually innocent until proven guilty, but out-of-control diabetes could well be a prime suspect in the following:

1. Vaginitis, specifically fungal in origin
2. Staphylococcal infections of the skin, such as boils, impetigo, and abscesses
3. Depression in states of both severe hyperglycemia and hypoglycemia
4. Changes of refractive error of the lens so that your glasses always seem too weak
5. Headaches (from hypoglycemia)
6. Insomnia and/or nightmares (from hypoglycemia)
7. Menstrual irregularities
8. Gum disease, which may lead to premature loss of teeth
9. High blood lipids (cholesterol, triglycerides)
10. Hypertension (high blood pressure)
11. Anemia
12. Decaying nails, specifically toenails
13. Necrobiosis diabeticorum (shin spots)
14. Osteoporosis (brittle bones)
15. Easy exhaustion from exercise or inability to achieve a training response to exercise. (Hyperglycemia does not let a muscle work; lactic acid builds up, and the pain prevents the person from continuing with the exercise. This stress causes the blood sugar to continue to rise and sets up a vicious cycle.)
16. Cataracts
17. Salivary-gland stones

June and Barbara: That's a long list of reasons to keep diabetes in control. Are there some other conditions that could be related to diabetes but that generally are not?

Dr. Jovanovic: That list is equally long, and it includes these conditions:

1. Itching
2. Headaches
3. Sinusitis
4. Vertigo
5. Tinnitus (a ringing in the ears)
6. Dizziness
7. Certain lung infections, including tuberculosis
8. Heart attacks
9. Gall-bladder disease and stones
10. Kidney and urine infections
11. Infertility
12. Hirsutism (excessive body and facial hair)
13. Amenorrhea (failure to menstruate)
14. Delayed puberty
15. Short stature
16. Contraction of joints
17. Neuropathy (more common from ingesting too much alcohol than from diabetes-related causes)

June and Barbara: If we ruled the world, even if we couldn't eliminate disease entirely, we'd at least make it only one to a customer. In other words, if you had one disease you couldn't get another. Is this rule already in effect in any way with diabetes? Is there any disease you're less likely to have if you have diabetes?

Dr. Jovanovic: Unfortunately, not to any extent. The only diseases I can think of that are less likely in diabetic women than in nondiabetic women are lupus erythematosus and sickle-cell anemia.

June and Barbara: Well, at least that's something. But let's go back to that point you made about the vast difference between in-control diabetes and out-of-control diabetes. Unfortunately, not all physicians make that distinction. When we were speaking at a diabetes conference at the Eisenhower Medical Center in Palm Desert, we listened to the physician speakers to learn more, as we always do. And as always, we heard again and again the dismal statistics about people with diabetes—how they're this percentage more likely to go blind and that percentage more likely to have kidney failure and the other percentage more likely to have one or more feet amputated.

June looked over at diabetic triathlete Bill Carlson, who was also in the audience. He was lean and fit and glowing with health. He'd been on a bike ride of 110 miles the day before and on his usual long-distance run that morning. What did these statistics have to do with him? And June considered herself and the fact that at her age she was in much better shape than all of her nondiabetic contemporaries and many of those ten or fifteen years younger. Her blood sugars were better than ever. (Practice makes perfect—well, *almost* perfect.) What did these statistics have to do with her? At dinner that night we discussed this situation. June theorized that there should now be two new categories of diabetes classification: Type C (for controlled) and Type U (for uncontrolled). They're really two different diseases with two different prognoses.

This reminded us of how angry our diabetic dietitian, Ron Brown, had been when he read somewhere the flat statement that diabetics don't heal well. "I heal as well as anybody," he growled. And so he does, because he's a Type C diabetic.

June also recalled that she'd been falsely diagnosed as having diabetic neuropathy by an orthopedist because he had noticed on her records that she was a diabetic. Did he ask her how her control was? No! He'd just assumed that since she was a diabetic, the predicted bad things were happening to her.

Our idea is that we should all work toward that happy day when every diabetic is either a Type IC or a Type IIC, with not a Type U to be seen. Then we'll never again have to listen to that dismal recitation of diabetes statistics. In pursuit of that goal, maybe you could tell us the control that we should shoot for (pun intended). We find that many of the diabetics we talk to—even some long-term diabetics—don't really know what their blood sugars should be. What constitutes the happy-medium condition known as euglycemia—not too high, not too low, but, like the baby bear's bed in the story of Goldilocks, just right?

Dr. Jovanovic: The answer to that is that the fasting or premeal blood sugar should be between 70 and 100; one hour after a meal, it should be 140; and two hours after a meal, it should be 120.

To achieve these blood sugars, which average 100 mg/dl, we allow the "swing" room to be down to 50 and up to 150, swinging around 100. This doesn't mean that we wouldn't decrease the insulin if the blood sugar were 50, but in the overall picture we accept these extremes.

June and Barbara: Do blood sugars vary from age to age? For example, are normal blood sugars for children different from normal blood sugars for adults?

Dr. Jovanovic: Yes, blood-sugar levels do vary with age. A newborn has a normal blood sugar of 40 to 60 mg/dl. Children ages one through five usually have fasting blood sugars of 60 mg/dl. Then, from eight to thirty years it stays at 70. After thirty years the fasting blood sugar goes up 1 mg/dl per year. So twenty years later, at the age of fifty, the normal fasting blood sugar is around 100 mg/dl. By the age of eighty, it may go to 130 mg/dl. This is all to say that the normal pancreas ages, and that as it does it gradually loses function.

June and Barbara: No matter what your age, of course, you want to be in good control. In order to achieve this goal, you have to know what your blood sugars are every day—in fact, several times a day—not just when you go to the doctor for an examination every three months or even once a month. Therefore, you have to be able to test your blood sugar yourself.

Ever since it came on the scene we've been passionate advocates of self-testing for blood sugar. June was doing it way back in 1978, when the only meter was the Ames Eyetone reflectance meter. The reason she got so excited about blood-sugar testing was that with the urine tests she always looked as if she were doing just fine, but when she started testing her blood sugar she was amazed and aghast to discover that even when her urine tests said she was normal, her blood sugar could be well over 200. Like many diabetic women over forty, she has a high renal threshold. This means that her kidneys don't spill sugar into her urine until her blood sugar is quite high, so according to the urine tests everything looked normal. Although in those days a meter cost $650 (they now cost around $150), June was determined to get one, because she knew it was the only way to know what was really happening to her blood sugar. (Luckily, she was able to find a used one for a reasonable price.)

June attributes the fact that she has absolutely no complications after twenty years of diabetes to two strategies: testing her blood sugar six or seven times a day, and taking appropriate action when her blood sugar is not normal. Do you feel as strongly as we do about the advantages of blood-sugar testing over urine testing?

Dr. Jovanovic: Absolutely. In explaining the difference between urine testing and blood-sugar testing to my patients, I like to use this automobile-speedometer analogy: Suppose you owned a car with a speedometer that was always way behind your actual driving speed—say, it would read thirty when you were actually going sixty miles an hour. Let's also say that the penalty for driving at sixty was life in prison. What would you do? You would surely get a new speedometer.

Such a lagging speedometer can be compared to testing your urine for sugar, when what you really need to know is the amount of sugar in your *blood* at any given moment. The sugar in your urine merely tells you about the sugar that was in your blood hours ago. Too late to prevent an arrest!

June and Barbara: Nevertheless, we still hear of physicians who have their patients test their urine along with their blood sugar. Do you feel there's any necessity for this?

Dr. Jovanovic: I usually don't play up urine tests, because I feel it distracts patients from blood-sugar tests. The only urine test I usually recommend is for ketones, which are substances formed during the metabolism of fat. When blood sugars are excessively high, the body converts its own fat into fuel. Ketones are released from fat cells when the cells break down from not having enough insulin in the bloodstream to hold them together. There are three fatty acids that are released from the fat cell. These three acids go to the liver, which converts them to ketones. A buildup of ketones makes the blood dangerously acidic.

June and Barbara: When is it important to test for ketones?

Dr. Jovanovic: I recommend it when the blood sugar is over 250.

June and Barbara: What should you do if you find you have ketones?

Dr. Jovanovic: Add one unit of regular insulin for every 25 mg/dl you are above 250. For instance, if you are 400 and there are ketones in your urine, take six units of regular insulin. Drink lots of water, and call the physician for further advice.

June and Barbara: Some women may hesitate to do their own blood-sugar testing because of the necessity of sticking your finger. We've seen women who calmly give themselves insulin injections two or three times a day but who are reluctant (and that's an understatement!) to start blood-sugar testing. Could you give them some reassurances?

Dr. Jovanovic: It's true that most women cringe at first at the thought of drawing their own blood to do the testing. It may be because of the memory of other times, when blood had to be drawn from the arm with a hypodermic needle and syringe, or when the finger actually had to be cut to let blood run out for other types of tests. But a large cut is no longer necessary. All it takes is a tiny pinprick, just enough to squeeze out one drop of blood. The pinprick heals almost immediately.

If a woman is worried that sticking her finger several times a day will make her fingertips ugly or scarred, she can look at the picture on page 31 of *The Diabetes Self-Care Method*, the book I coauthored with Dr. Charles Peterson. The picture is a close-up of four fingertips without a mark on them. The caption reads, "These are the tips of the fingers of a diabetic person who, for the past eight years, has monitored her own blood glucose. During this time, she measured her blood glucose seven or more times per day. Taking a blood sample from her fingers

20,000 times has not ruined the appearance of her hands, as you can see, but it has certainly aided in diabetes control." Those fingertips are mine.

There are a number of small automatic finger-sticking devices on the market now. These move so quickly that you probably won't feel a thing. Another way to eliminate pain in blood-sugar testing is to stick the sides of your fingers rather than the tips. The tips have more nerves and thus a greater sensitivity to pain. The blood flow is also better on the sides of the fingers than on the fingertips. You can demonstrate this by squeezing the side of your forefinger with your other thumb and forefinger. The pinched area gets quite pink, indicating the presence of blood. You won't see that to the same degree if you pinch the tips.

To get the kind of nice, large drop of blood you need for the test, you should let your arm hang down below the level of your heart after sticking the side of your finger. Then you "milk" the finger until you can squeeze out enough blood to cover the pad on the test strip. Try to let the blood flow onto the pad; don't smear it or rub it on. You want a shiny drop of blood that sits up on the pad.

Let the blood remain on the pad for the appropriate period of time (it will differ for different test strips). Then wipe or blot the blood off (this part of the technique also differs with different strips). Some strips are then read visually by comparing the colors to the colors on the side of the strip container. Others can be read only in blood-sugar meters. Still others can be read both ways.

Regardless of which method you prefer to use, the important thing is that you're able to know from such self-testing whether your blood sugar is high, normal, or low. You can then immediately take the necessary steps to correct the situation or report abnormal blood sugars to your doctor, who can help you change your therapy to keep your blood sugars in the normal range.

June and Barbara: We're glad you brought out the purpose of blood-sugar testing. We've come across a number of people at the Sugarfree Center who lose sight of what it's really for. They're the victims of a strange new disease that we've come to call the bad-meter syndrome. Here's how it works: After deciding that reading strips visually is not precise and accurate enough, a diabetic person carefully looks over all the available meters, selects one, and receives instruction in its use. She then takes it home and starts testing. It may look as though she's testing her blood sugar, but she's really testing the *meter*, trying to prove it wrong. She may take a blood sugar on the meter and back it up with a visual reading on a Chemstrip, Glucostix, or Visidex strip. She then decides she can tell from the visual reading (the same visual reading that she previously thought imprecise and inaccurate) that the meter is off.

She may do five or six blood sugars in a row and see the numbers rise or fall, which convinces her that the meter is useless. In reality it's quite possible for blood sugar to fall rapidly and rise rapidly (especially when you're angry or disturbed or frustrated). June was demonstrating a meter to a young woman whose blood sugar went up 45 mg/dl in five minutes in response to her fear of having her finger punctured.

Or the diabetic may take a blood sugar on her meter in the doctor's office or a lab to see if they come out the same. If the results are different, as is usually the case, the patient then says, "Aha! The meter *is* bad!!"

Or the meter may indicate that she has an unusually high or low blood sugar, and she can't figure out why.

She decides that she can't have a blood sugar that high or low; the meter must be wrong.

We'll admit that on rare occasions there is something wrong with the meter, but the Ames Technical Service reported that 90 percent of the meters returned to them as defective were working perfectly. A meter problem is usually shown by its failure to work at all or by strange flashings or buzzings, not by its just being a few (or several) points off in reading. More often, especially when you take repeated blood sugars within a short period of time and they differ widely, it's a matter of inconsistent operator technique. You can only gain consistency through lots of calm and careful practice.

Differences can also be caused by using capillary blood at home and venous blood in the office or lab. Capillary whole blood is 15 percent lower than the venous plasma blood. Also, we have a feeling that the lab is sometimes wrong. In your experience, Dr. Jovanovic, are the lab tests always accurate?

Dr. Jovanovic: Not at all. When I checked the lab at my hospital, it was off by 15 percent half the time, and the direction of the error was random.

June and Barbara: How do you make sure the lab tests you're dealing with are accurate?

Dr. Jovanovic: I prefer to double-check the home blood-glucose monitors rather than check labs. I sometimes use what you might call human control. I have the patient take the fasting blood sugar of a nondiabetic family member. If a person doesn't have diabetes, it's remarkable how perfect the numbers will be—70 to 80 mg/dl will be the answer 90 percent of the time. If that's the reading on the meter, then the patient can rely on the meter for her own blood sugars. In addition to this human control, I also keep in my office standard control solutions (I call them play blood) made by each meter company to double-check all my patients' machines.

June and Barbara: Yes, we urge people to use these control solutions, too. Since they're set at a known glucose level, you can check both your meter's accuracy and your own technique by seeing whether you can make your meter read the control solution within an acceptable range. There's even a new control fluid on the market, Sugar-Chex, that can be used in almost all the home meters and the lab machines, so it's possible to check them all out against each other with it.

We're both distressed and pleased that you mentioned the inaccuracy of lab blood tests. We're distressed because it would be a comfort to know that there's one test you can absolutely rely on. But we're also pleased to be vindicated. We've had people stomp into the Sugar-free Center in high dudgeon because their lab test didn't agree with their meter reading. When we run every possible kind of control solution and test on the meter and repeatedly show that the meter is reading accurately, they still won't believe it. The lab result is the only thing that counts with them, and, as you point out, they're frequently putting their faith in a weak vessel. As in most areas of life, it winds up that you have to trust yourself and your own controls and test results.

Despite the fact that it is terribly expensive and time-consuming to keep running unnecessary tests, bad-meter syndrome would otherwise be harmless except for one thing: you lose your perspective. We've seen people all wild and hysterical because their "bad" meter read their blood sugar as only 264, while the lab read it at 282. They're not upset over the fact that their blood sugar is over 200. No, they're only upset with the meter. The president of one of the companies manufacturing meters said he had an irate phone call from a diabetic complaining because the meter "only" read up to 399. Although he had broken the bank on the meter with his high blood sugar, he didn't seem to want to do anything about it. He just wanted to get mad at the meter for not giving him even higher numbers.

Certainly, you want an accurate meter—but unless something really wild is going on, you should relax. All of the meters are basically accurate (within $\pm$ 10 percent), or the FDA wouldn't have given approval for them to be on the market. It's true that there may be an occasional off-reading, but that can be the fault of an off-strip or an off-operator or even an unclean machine. We shudder at the filthy, mucky state of some of the meters that we saw come in during a trade-in program. Some of them even came in from hospitals.

Of course, we realize that people often displace their anger at diabetes, directing it instead toward something more acceptable, like their meter, the doctor, or the doctor's bills. But if this displacement causes you to lose sight of the goal of good control, it can be detrimental to your health.

In the final analysis you should put your concern where it belongs, on keeping your blood sugar in the normal range. The meter is only a means to that end, only a messenger delivering the news. Don't follow in that inglorious tradition of killing the messenger who delivers bad news.

Another important test for assaying your control is the glycosylated-hemoglobin, or hemoglobin A_1C, test. Many women haven't heard of this at all and others have only a vague idea of what it is, of who needs it, and of what the results should be. Can you help us with that?

Dr. Jovanovic: In the early sixties a blood banker noted that 5 percent of the donors had an elevation of a component of hemoglobin that was barely present in the other 95 percent of the population. He then noted that these individuals were the same persons who had diabetes. He concluded from this that there is a genetic marker for diabetes. It was not until the mid-seventies that it was learned that it is the sugar in the blood of diabetic persons that modifies hemoglobin to A_1C, and not diabetes *per se.*

Thus, hemoglobin A_1C is a modified component of hemoglobin A (which is the majority of hemoglobin in our blood). The higher the blood-glucose level, the more hemoglobin A becomes hemoglobin A_1C. The reaction is essentially irreversible, and once hemoglobin A_1C is formed it stays formed for the life span of the red-blood cell (about 120 days).

The formula is: hemoglobin A + sugar yields hemoglobin A_1C.

The hemoglobin A_1C test can be used as a retrospect scope in that the amount of hemoglobin A_1C is directly related to the glucose levels over time. While the on rate for sugar onto hemoglobin A is rapid, the off rate is slow. In other words, it is more sensitive to sin than to repentance. The on rate is one to two weeks of high blood-glucose levels; the off rate is six weeks to two months.

The test is simple in that it does not require the woman to be fasting, since it is not affected by the moment-to-moment variations of blood glucose. Neither is it very sensitive to minor changes in blood glucose: in order for the hemoglobin A_1C to be raised by 1 percent, the blood-sugar average needs to be 20 mg/dl higher. The normal range varies from laboratory to laboratory. Thus, a woman should not only ask what the result of her test is but also what is normal for the particular laboratory.

Glycosylated hemoglobin cannot be used to make

the diagnosis of diabetes, as it is not sensitive enough. This diagnosis can only be made through a glucose-tolerance test.

As a monitor of glucose levels over time, an A_1C is good for about two months. Therefore, as a double check on a woman's diabetes program, A_1C tests should be taken no farther apart than every three months. This frequency in checking allows for intervention before prolonged periods of high blood-glucose levels take their toll.

June and Barbara: A woman who had a rather dismal experience with her diabetes while in the hospital wants to know what you can do to maintain your control when the nurses and doctors take over and seem to be making your blood sugars bounce around in a very scary way, not to mention the fact that the food that arrives on your tray is often too much of the wrong thing. In fact, we constantly hear stories from experienced diabetic women about traumatic hospital stays.

Dr. Jovanovic: What happens is that education is a blessing in disguise, for the more you know, the more frustrating it is to be treated inappropriately. All of my well-educated patients find themselves in situations in which they know more than the health-care team. There are several positive results of this potentially anxiety-provoking situation. First, become a gentle teacher and explain that you measure your own blood sugar and that it helps you to decide your own doses of insulin. Consequently, you need access to your meter and insulin. The physician in charge should be able to help you get permission to continue to do self-care, even though you are in a hospital.

Second, allow the staff to test your meter if they are not sure of its accuracy. They want to see how close you can get to the lab result. If you can accurately measure your sugar, you have proven that you can use your meter skillfully, and this demonstration will usually stop the blood-drawing team from sticking you!

Third, if things are not exactly the way you want, allow for a bit of flexibility. Usually their way is not so bad.

Finally, above all remember that you still have rights as a citizen and can refuse anything that does not seem right.

As far as my own stories go, it is amazing to me that I have had the dumb luck of consistent mishaps. But it doesn't happen just to me. My six-year-old daughter was in the hospital to have an orthopedic procedure performed on her left leg. The surgeon came by and picked up her right leg and said, "We'll have this leg perfect again in the morning." My daughter told him that her right leg was perfect and she wanted her *left* leg fixed! I was so worried that I wrote "Fix this one" across her left leg as they took her off to the operating room. The moral of the story is that you should be assertive—if something is not right, speak out!

June and Barbara: We received a letter containing a specific question that may actually turn out to be a more general one: "About eleven years after developing diabetes, I developed a thyroid condition known as Graves' disease. My doctor did not think it was related to my diabetes, but a year later I read an article in the *ADA Forecast* that said that thyroid conditions do seem to be somehow related to diabetes. Do women seem more prone to this than men?"

Dr. Jovanovic: Forty percent of all Type I patients have a coexisting thyroid disease. This is presumably based on the same antibody attack on the thyroid as on the pancreas. Other glands that can also be attacked are the adrenal, ovary, pituitary, and parathyroids, as well as the stomach lining, which produces B_{12}. For this reason all diabetic women should be checked periodically for the status of these glands.

June and Barbara: Some women have complained about leg cramps. Do you know what causes these and what they can do about them?

Dr. Jovanovic: Leg cramps tend to happen to all people, men or women, diabetic persons or nondiabetic persons. However, with large swings in blood glucose, other ions such as sodium, potassium, and calcium, which because of their chemical properties of positive charge are called *cations,* also tend to swing. Leg cramps are the result of these cationic fluxes. The blood levels of these cations do not reflect their muscle levels. There are many causes of cationic disturbances at the muscle level, among them:

chronic diuretic therapy with muscle potassium loss, extremes of calcium intake—too little for a long time or too much for a long time—and
stasis, which can be caused by sitting too long, wearing high boots or knee-high hose, having varicose veins, or being pregnant (which can stop the blood return from the legs).

The best treatment is to replace potassium losses, normalize calcium intake, avoid wearing knee-highs or high boots, avoid sitting for longer than an hour without raising the legs, give birth, and—last but not least—do stretching exercises before bed. If the muscle is stretched before bed, it will have less of a tendency to cramp up. My favorite exercise is to stand four to five feet from the wall and then lean into it, holding the position while I watch the 11 P.M. news.

June and Barbara: We had an inquiry from a woman in her forties, an artist and photographer who does quite strenuous gymnastics. She wanted to know about microalbumin—specifically, why it appears in the urine after heavy workouts and whether it leads to kidney disease.

Dr. Jovanovic: Exercise increases cardiac output. As the blood rushes past the kidney, albumin—a small molecular-weight protein—is filtered into the urine. Albumin usually does not appear in the urine unless the pressure is increased, as is the case with strenuous exercise. Microalbuminuria, or albumin in the urine, is a normal response to strenuous exercise. Albumin is also lost when the kidney has been damaged because of diabetes, causing the filter to become "leaky." Although both situations produce albumin in the urine, exercise does not increase the leak from diabetic nephropathy.

June and Barbara: Apparently her gymnastics aren't doing her any harm, then. But are there some sports and exercise a diabetic woman should avoid?

Dr. Jovanovic: The only sports that should be avoided pertain to women with diabetic retinopathy. Any exercise that places the head below the heart is thought to increase pressure in the eye and perhaps lead to bleeding in the retina.

June and Barbara: Would weight-lifting and/or strenuous high-impact aerobic dancing also be bad for someone with retinopathy?

Dr. Jovanovic: Yes, this too would raise pressure in the eye. Consult with your eye doctor if you have retinopathy so that he or she can help you plan a safe exercise program.

Of course, a diabetic woman should check her blood sugar before any exercise session to ensure that she does not have a hypoglycemic episode during the session. A well-controlled woman should exercise with her blood glucose at 70–150 mg/dl and should check her blood sugar every twenty minutes to make sure it isn't dropping.

June and Barbara: A woman wrote us that she was disturbed about the unusual amount of facial hair she had developed and wondered whether her diabetes was causing this.

Dr. Jovanovic: Once upon a time a teacher of mine in medical school announced that he could always tell a woman with diabetes by whether she had a moustache. I immediately became alarmed, for I always thought that my subtle upper-lip hairs were there because of my Mediterranean background. His statement haunted me, and I then began scrutinizing the upper lip of all my diabetic female patients. My professor was clearly wrong—not all diabetic women have moustaches. But a lot of them do.

Then about five years ago I read an article on the increased prevalence of hirsutism (overgrowth of hair) in women with a long duration of diabetes. The article claimed that prolonged use of insulin is associated with elevations in the male hormone, testosterone, which stimulates facial-hair growth. However, not all faces have numerous potential hair follicles. Therefore, the testosterone would have no effect on hair growth in a fair-skinned Scandinavian woman, whereas a dark-haired lass like me tends to have hair growth.

If the testosterone level is up for any reason, hair will grow. For example, testosterone levels are normally highest at the time of ovulation, and many women note that they need to shave more frequently during this time than any other time of the month.

There is a form of diabetes—overweight Type II—that has markedly elevated insulin levels because of severe insulin resistance. These high levels of insulin thicken the outer coating of the ovary and cause it to turn into a testosterone factory. If these women have the genetic tendency toward dark hair follicles on their faces, they will grow more hair.

The treatment of hairiness includes both decreasing the testosterone level and destroying the hair follicles with electrolysis.

June and Barbara: One jet-set businesswoman wrote to ask if she would have any problem taking her meter and strips through an airport security X-ray machine. We contacted all the meter manufacturers and received the information that none of the meters or strips would be damaged by airport X-ray machines. These meters and strips include the Glucometer I and II, Dextrostix, and Glucostix; Accu-Chek bG and II and Chemstrips; Glucoscan Plus, 2000, and 3000 and Glucoscan Strips; Glucochek II and SC; Diascan and Diascan Strips; and TrendsMeter and TrendsStrips.

A couple of the manufacturers said that if you wanted to be 100 percent certain of no damage, the meter and strips could be placed in one of the leaded bags used for film. However, they reiterated that such a step really isn't necessary.

June has sometimes been stopped by airport security because of the jet injector, which does look something like a small torpedo. But after she explains what it is, they simply wave her through.

As a jet-setter in your own right, Dr. Jovanovic, winging to diabetes conferences all over the world, have you any travel tips?

Dr. Jovanovic: I would like to comment on airline food. The airlines make one generic sick tray. This is an all-purpose meal for everyone with some kind of ailment, be it peptic-ulcer disease, high blood pressure, kidney disease, or diabetes. Consequently, it is bland, saltless, sugarless, and tasteless.

In addition, when the flight attendant asks over the loudspeaker, "Will the diabetic please identify herself?" I can't bring myself to push the call button to be singled out. I would much rather pick and choose from a normal tray. If the meal is composed of too many forbidden foods, my carry-on has a supply of supplements.

Sometimes when I have a choice, I fly after dinner. From 8 P.M. onward, the airlines do not generally serve meals.

June and Barbara: Diabetic women often report that they keep having mood swings. Is this due to hypoglycemia or hyperglycemia?

Dr. Jovanovic: Both! Hypoglycemia may be subtle and can present itself as anger or depression. Hyperglycemia may show itself as anxiety, irritability, and/or unstable emotions. Improved glucose control improves mood, and improved mood improves glucose control.

June and Barbara: Since diabetes is a blood-sugar disorder, we often get questions on another blood-sugar disorder, hypoglycemia—not as a condition occurring in diabetes but as a separate disease in the nondiabetic population. People who have it—or think they have it—probably come to us because they have nowhere else to turn. Another reason they seek us out is that hypoglycemia is sometimes a precursor of diabetes. Sometimes going to the doctor doesn't help much, because many physicians seem to fall into one of two camps. There are those who think hypoglycemia as a separate disease doesn't even exist. And there are others—far, far fewer in number—who seem to think that everybody has it and that it's responsible for all the world's evils, including most of the crime, from minor juvenile delinquency to murder. Remember the famous trial of former San Francisco supervisor Dan White, who was accused of murdering the mayor and another supervisor? His lawyer presented what came to be known as the Twinkie defense, in which he explained that White was out of control of the situation because he'd been eating so much junk food—including Twinkies—which presumably gave him hypoglycemia.

Even war has been blamed on low blood sugar. We've heard reports of a particularly warlike South American tribe, all the members of which are vegetarians. One hypothesis is that because of the lack of protein in their diet these people always have low blood sugar, and that this is what makes them so belligerent.

At any rate, the truth about hypoglycemia must lie somewhere between total nonexistence and a widespread cult disease. Could you shed some light on what it really is—and isn't?

Dr. Jovanovic: Hypoglycemia is defined as a below-normal blood-glucose level. The question of what a normal blood-glucose level is has been debated over the years. The controversy finally seems to be settled now that we've learned that in various stages of life there are different levels of normal. See the discussion of normal ranges by age earlier in this chapter.

Young, lean persons tend to drift down to 40 mg/dl if they have not eaten for two to four hours. Their normal, healthy pancreases secrete insulin to match the food ingested. Typically, these young people have only juice and toast for breakfast. This is a pure-carbohydrate meal. The normal pancreas would secrete large amounts of insulin to ensure that the blood-glucose level does not rise. The carbohydrate in this meal metabolizes within one hour. The insulin secreted hangs around for three hours, despite the fact that the food has disappeared, and it drives down the blood sugar because there's no leftover food in the bloodstream to work on. Thus, three hours after a pure-carbohydrate meal these people are ravenously hungry, have headaches, and feel irritable and shaky. Their blood glucose is around 40. This reaction is called reactive hypoglycemia and is completely normal. The situation can be prevented by eating a breakfast that is not composed solely of carbohydrates, but also includes fat and protein. The fat in this mixed meal slows down the carbohydrate absorption to allow it to stay around longer. Protein metabolizes to sugars in two or three hours after you eat and is thus a perfect buffer for the residual insulin in the bloodstream at the three-hour point.

It's estimated that 40 percent of all lean persons go down to 40 mg/dl blood sugar if they don't eat for four hours after a pure-carbohydrate meal. Therefore, reactive hypoglycemia is a normal response, but that doesn't make it any less uncomfortable to experience.

June and Barbara: We often suggest that people check themselves to see if those symptoms you describe actually are the result of low blood sugar. Rather than having to go to the doctor for an expensive glucose-tolerance test, they can get a can of Chemstrips, cut these in half vertically (thereby getting two for the price of one), and take their blood sugar using an inexpensive lancing device whenever they have those strange feelings.

Dr. Jovanovic: Yes, and if they find that their blood sugar is low at those times, they can then "cure" the disease merely by changing the menu. The following is a recommended meal plan for treating reactive hypoglycemia.

1. No concentrated sweets—no cakes, candies, sugars, cookies, and so on.
2. All carbohydrates eaten should be complex and high in fiber to delay absorption—for example, oats, brown rice, celery, bran, lentils, and beans.
3. The carbohydrates should make up less than 40 percent of the total daily calorie requirement. The rest should be 30–40 percent protein, and the remaining calories are fat.
4. There should be three meals and four snacks every day. The distribution of calories should be as follows:

   Breakfast: 20 percent
   Midmorning snack: 5 percent
   Lunch: 30 percent
   Afternoon snack: 5 percent
   Dinner: 30 percent
   Early evening snack: 5 percent
   Bedtime snack: 5 percent

   The best snacks are high in protein (for example, milk, cheese, and meat).
5. To prevent weight gain, the total calories consumed each day should be less than 12 per pound of weight. For a 110-pound woman, this is around 1250 calories a day.

June and Barbara: We seem to find more women—particularly young women—than men complaining of hypoglycemia.

Dr. Jovanovic: Young women, perhaps depressed and emotionally needy, can receive secondary gain from finding an illness to use as a crutch by which they can be dependent on others. It's possible that some physicians have taken advantage of these needs, ordering numerous expensive tests that required many visits and concocting injections to relieve the symptoms. One treatment that used to be popular was known as adrenal extract. This treatment did nothing medically, but psychologically it exerted wondrous powers. Societies and clubs even sprang up in which sufferers could commiserate with one another.

June and Barbara: If this reactive hypoglycemia is a normal condition that can be corrected with diet, is there any kind of hypoglycemia that is abnormal and that requires serious medical intervention?

Dr. Jovanovic: Fasting hypoglycemia is not normal. Less than 5 percent of all persons who suffer from hypoglycemia have it happen in the fasting state. If a person spontaneously suffers from falling blood-glucose levels, there may be a very real and dangerous underlying disease. The causes of spontaneous hypoglycemia include:

1. Hormonal deficiencies. Children and pregnant women will manifest profound hypoglycemia if they lose adrenal function for any reason. Nonpregnant adults do not become hypoglycemic if their adrenal glands fail.
2. Infection and severe malnutrition. When people in Third World countries with severe famine catch an infection, they can have profound hypoglycemia. Infections that have been reported to do this are malaria, cholera, and tuberculosis.
3. Drug ingestion. If a nondiabetic person takes insulin or sulfonylureal agents, hypoglycemia will ensue. Of course, persons with diabetes can become hypoglycemic if they take too much insulin or sulfonylureal agent and/or do not eat their prescribed meal, and/or exercise more than usual.

4. Tumors (affects less than 1 percent of hypoglycemia sufferers).

    a. Insulinoma. This is a tumor in the pancreas that secretes insulin in large quantities regardless of the food ingested. The tumor must be removed surgically to prevent life-threatening hypoglycemia. These tumors are often numerous and so small that the surgeon needs to take out almost all of the pancreas in order to look for the tumor under the microscope.

    b. Other cancers that secrete insulin-like hormones. Here, too, the tumors need to be removed to prevent life-threatening hypoglycemia. Typically, cancers that have been reported to secrete insulin-like hormones include melanoma, sarcoma, adenocarcinoma, and lymphoma.

Hypoglycemia, no matter what the cause, no matter whether in a diabetic person or not, manifests itself as irritability, slowing of the ability to think, slurred speech, confusion, tremor, chill, and, if profound low blood sugar occurs, the result is coma and then death. (Remember the cases of the "insulin killers"?) Given all of this, it's no wonder that the word *hypoglycemia* is so charged with emotion.

June and Barbara: We've heard that hypoglycemia can be the precursor of diabetes and that people with hypoglycemia are very likely to later become diabetic. Is this so?

Dr. Jovanovic: There is no evidence that people who go down to 40 mg/dl four hours after they have eaten pure carbohydrate are more likely to get diabetes. It is true, however, that people who have a high blood sugar one hour after a meal (with *high* defined as over 200 mg/dl) and who then "crash" from 200 down to 40 do have a higher risk of diabetes, perhaps double the risk of people in the general population.

June and Barbara: We've heard of two kinds of diets recommended for people with a tendency toward reactive hypoglycemia. One is high protein and the other is high complex carbohydrate, high fiber, and low fat. An example of the latter is Dr. James Anderson's HCF diet, which has also been used for diabetic women. Do you have any preferences with these?

Dr. Jovanovic: In my opinion the best way to avoid reactive hypoglycemia is to eat mixed meals, mostly high in fiber content, and to have adequate protein and fat in meals. I would definitely recommend a consultation with a dietitian in order to learn food composition and meal planning, as well as to get assistance in setting up a diet that is both helpful in avoiding reactive hypoglycemia and compatible with your taste in food.

June and Barbara: In days gone by, a woman's role was defined as that of *Kinder, Kirche, Küche*—children, church, and cooking. While the modern woman certainly isn't confined to these three, we have noticed in the questions we receive that many women still seem to be the defenders of the faith and tend to worry more than men about possible conflicts between their religion and their diabetes care.

For example, a diabetes nurse educator got in touch with us because she was concerned about a patient who was an insulin-taking diabetic woman. The patient was a member of the Christian Science church and was planning to take a trip with friends who were members of the same church. Her friends didn't know that this woman was a diabetic person, and she didn't plan to tell them because she was ashamed of taking insulin, feeling it showed a lack of faith. The nurse was worried that if the woman had a reaction, no one would know what was going on and they wouldn't know how to help her.

We wrote to the board of directors of the First Church of Christ, Scientist in Boston and received a thoughtful response from the manager of the committees on publication. It is such a lucid and caring letter that we recommend that anyone who may be wrestling with such a decision read it in entirety (if you write to us at the Sugarfree Center, we'll be glad to send you a copy). We would like to include this brief excerpt here:

> As for guilt feelings, I don't think these ordinarily would (or should) be a problem for a Christian Scientist who has decided to seek medical help. The teachings of Christian Science simply do not point a condemning finger at such individuals, much less equate sickness simplistically with "lack of faith." Nor does the church encourage the view that those who use medicine are somehow committing a sin. A Christian Scientist who turns to a doctor in [a] difficult circumstance would be less apt to dwell on feelings of failure than to resolve all the more to work and pray for the spiritual understanding and closeness to God that is, we believe, the ultimate source for freedom and healing. This would be as true in the case of someone electing to use insulin for an indefinite period as it would be in any other situation.

On another occasion, an Orthodox Jewish woman was concerned about using pork insulin. This time we contacted the Los Angeles Board of Rabbis, who quoted from the *Practical Medical Halacha:* "There is no prohibition against deriving benefit from nonkosher animals. The prohibition against eating nonkosher foods does not apply to injectables. Hence, all types of insulin, whether derived from beef or pork or other nonkosher sources, may be used without any halachic concern."

In your practice, have you ever come across problems of religion or philosophy in conflict with diabetes control—for example, a person who wanted to fast for religious reasons?

Dr. Jovanovic: Yes, this has happened. Fortunately, the Jewish law exempts pregnant and nursing women from fasting. So far, most of my patients' fasting has not been a problem, but we have had to make some very clever maneuvers with insulin to allow for Jewish ritualistic foods, such as matzo (a very high-carbohydrate, unleavened bread), Manischewitz wine (which is sweeter than grape juice), and honey and apples, which are a customary part of welcoming the New Year.

A greater challenge is the Indian diet, which is devoid of meat and is 70 percent carbohydrate. All these special situations require changes in insulin, but so far we seem to have found ways to keep the religion *and* to keep the sugar controlled.

June and Barbara: On the other hand, following the tenets of certain religions can be a positive factor in diabetes. The *American Journal of Public Health* proposed the thesis that a vegetarian diet reduces the risk of developing diabetes. Based on a twenty-one-year study of a population of 25,698 white adult Seventh-Day Adventists (most of whom follow a vegetarian diet) diabetes was found to be the underlying cause of death in the men of this faith at half the rate that diabetes causes death in all U.S. white males.

While we're on this subject, June demands equal time for Buddhism, which is as much a philosophy as a religion. We find that diabetics and those who work with diabetics are well advised to strive for the four Buddhist virtues: joy, friendliness, compassion, and equanimity. This last word has a richness of meaning. The dictionary defines it as "emotional or mental stability or composure, especially under tension or strain; calmness, equilibrium." Think what developing these virtues would do for controlling your diabetes and enhancing your life!

And here's a Buddhist thought that could apply equally well to diabetes and to any other adversity you may be called upon to face: Bless your enemy, for he enables you to grow.

CHAPTER
2
AGES AND STAGES

They order the matter of ages and stages better in France than in the United States. Take, for example, the Miss/Mrs. controversy that we've tried—for the most part unsuccessfully—to resolve with the hybrid Ms. In France there's no problem. You're Mademoiselle until you marry or reach that indeterminate *un certain âge* at which time you automatically become Madame.

Then there's the nomenclatural wrestling that we do in this country when referring to people who are, shall we say, mature. We've tried "senior citizen" (ugh!) and "the elderly," both of which conjure up visions of decrepitude, and we've also tried such euphemisms as "the golden years." In France, there is no problem—this stage of life is called simply and straightforwardly *le troisième âge* (the third age).

In keeping with this, and following an *Alice in Wonderland* admonition, "Speak in French, remember who you are," we're going to divide the woman diabetic's ages and stages into *le premier âge, le deuxième âge,* and *le troisième âge.* In the first of these we'll discuss childhood and puberty to the extent that as far as diabetes is concerned, these ages differ for girls and young women in comparison to those of the masculine persuasion. Because we did not receive many questions from children, adolescents, or their parents, and neither June nor Lois nor Barbara has a diabetic child, in this section we will deal primarily with type I diabetes in general. It's this type that generally appears during the first third of life.

In *le deuxième âge,* we'll cover the events that usually occur in this period: career choices, marriage, and pregnancy.

In *le* good old *troisième âge,* we'll not only go into the significant physiological and psychological aspects of menopause but we'll also explore Type II diabetes, both generally and specifically, because the majority of cases of this type of diabetes come to light during this period of life.

And so, *Mademoiselles* and *Mesdames,* let's get to it, or, in other words, *allons-y.*

Le Premier Âge

Gail Sheehy, writing in her book *The Spirit of Survival,* says:

> Sudden or disorienting change introduced into the family or social and political environment of a child does not necessarily leave permanent scars on the temperament. Quite the contrary. Adversity is part of life, and learning to master adversity is one of the basic ways of gaining self-confidence and self-esteem. Disorders of behavior that may develop while a child or adolescent is in the midst of a crisis often subside or disappear once a

consistency of environment and relationships is reestablished. And the experience of knowing one has survived can offer a psychological shield against future disasters in adult life.

We were discussing this with Dr. Jovanovic and she echoed Gail Sheehy's sentiment. "I truly believe," she said, "that behind every great woman is a child who has had to suffer in one way or another."

We all agree, however, that there's no point in just suffering for suffering's sake. Therefore, in this section we'll try to present information that will keep suffering at a minimum for the diabetic girl and Type I woman and develop coping skills that will minimize diabetes problems.

We cannot here go into every aspect of being or raising a diabetic child. That would fill an entire book on its own. In fact, it would fill *three* books—those by Lee Ducat, Mimi Belmonte, M.D., and Gloria Loring described in Appendix A. We recommend these books to every mother of a diabetic child and to every young diabetic reader.

June and Barbara: We've heard some mothers of diabetic babies and very small children say that they prefer to do urine tests because they can't bear to stick the little fingers. Do you think that it's okay to substitute urine tests in this case?

Dr. Jovanovic: No. The smaller the child, the more important it is to know what the blood sugar is immediately. Hypoglycemia presents itself in peculiar ways in infants, especially ones who do not talk yet.

June and Barbara: Given the smallness of their fingers, how often do you think children this little should have blood sugars taken?

Dr. Jovanovic: Even if their fingers are small, they do have ten of them—and ten toes as well—so there are sufficient places from which to take the blood samples. I feel that at least three times a day is not too often for infants and small children to have blood-sugar tests.

June and Barbara: Do you believe that it's a good idea for diabetic girls and teenagers to attend special diabetes camps?

Dr. Jovanovic: Yes, yes, a thousand times yes! I don't know how many times I have had young women tell me that they felt terribly alone as adolescents. Diabetes embarrassed them so they hid it; rather than sleeping over at a girlfriend's house and risk being found out, they chose to be alone.

The camp experience is wonderful. The campers, and even most of the counselors, have diabetes. The child immediately feels part of the majority. Insulin therapy, diet, and the camp experience are all molded into one. Once a camper learns how to adjust the diet and insulin to compensate for the track meet, the swimming competition, the campout, and the hike, then she's ready for a camp that does not specialize in diabetes.

Simply asking a regular camp to "watch out" for a diabetic child is inviting the child to a summer of chance —the chance that nothing bad will happen. There are more than thirty camps in America for diabetic children (see Appendix B). Surely one would fit any child's special interests and still be a place where diabetes skills can be reinforced.

June and Barbara: We especially agree with how important it is for the diabetic child to feel part of the majority for a change. We think that's good for diabetics of all ages. Since we have so many diabetic employees and all of the clients at our Sugarfree Centers are diabetics, a *non*diabetic can feel a little awkward and out of place. Whenever Barbara is talking to our clients there and they ask, with a hopeful smile, "Are *you* a diabetic?" she always looks down in embarrassment, scuffs her toe against the carpet, and has to admit, "Well, no, actually I'm not." But she adds, quickly, "I try to live as if I am one, though!" She says that in these situations she feels like the outcast member of a certain tribe in South America in which almost everyone has a goiter because of a lack of iodine, a genetic trait, or both. When a child, through some quirk of nature, does not develop a goiter, his little friends taunt him, saying things like "Nyah, nyah, bottleneck."

Dr. Jovanovic: It's good for everybody to have these reverse experiences from time to time in order to see how the other half feels.

June and Barbara: When a young girl begins to menstruate, does this affect her diabetes in any way?

Dr. Jovanovic: With the beginning of menstruation or puberty, control of blood sugars usually deteriorates—as reflected by rising glycosylated hemoglobin levels—even though the doctors tend to increase insulin doses. In fact, unstable diabetes is a common problem in young patients with Type I diabetes, particularly during adolescence.

This deterioration of control is usually blamed on the psychosocial upheavals in an adolescent's life or on cheating on the diet. However, a study by Stephanie Amiel recently published in the *New England Journal of Medicine* clearly showed that it is the high levels of maturation hormones that cause the diabetes to be out of control if the insulin dose is not doubled.

Thus, puberty is a time when the insulin dose needs to be adjusted upward. The largest dose of insulin tends to be the overnight insulin dose, because the highest secretion of growth hormone and the sex hormones is at the point of deepest sleeping. Since growth hormone and the sex hormones are anti-insulin in action, the insulin dose of necessity needs to be adjusted upward.

One mystery is why diabetic complications never occur before puberty, no matter how many years the diabetes has existed. It is almost as though the complications time clock doesn't start ticking off the years until after the onset of menstruation. It is hoped that tight control may stop this clock.

June and Barbara: We've had a lot of questions from women who find that their blood sugar goes up unexpectedly just before the onset of their menstrual period. (Actually, it isn't unexpected, since it happens every month!) Is this a common occurrence?

Dr. Jovanovic: Yes. It's quite usual for blood sugars to go up markedly between two and five days before the menstrual period.

June and Barbara: Why is this?

Dr. Jovanovic: Throughout the course of the menstrual cycle, levels of various hormones in a woman's body change drastically. Let me review for you the normal menstrual cycle to make clear what happens and when.

The normal cycle has two phases. The first, or follicular, phase has its onset on day one, coincident with the onset of menses. During this first phase, the female hormones—specifically, estrogen and progesterone—are at their lowest levels. These two hormones exert an action against insulin. Thus, when their levels are low, insulin seems stronger. In other words, less insulin is required to keep the blood sugar normal, even if food intake is not altered.

By day fourteen, or midway through the cycle, the

pituitary releases another hormone, luteinizing hormone (LH), which causes an egg (ovum) to be released from the ovary. This starts the second, or luteal, phase of the cycle. The egg then travels down a tube (the fallopian tube) to the womb (uterus).

Meanwhile, the egg's old wrappings in the ovary turn into a hormone factory (corpus luteum) and secrete large quantities of estrogen and progesterone to prepare the uterine lining (endometrium) for the nestling-in of the ovum if the ovum perchance meets its counterpart, the sperm, swimming up the tube. In this chance encounter, if the ovum and sperm are united (conception), they arrive as one unit (the trophoblast) to take up housekeeping in the warm, boggy, prepared endometrium.

If the ovum is not fertilized, it will not nestle into the endometrium but will merely wash out of the vagina. The corpus luteum, which produced the estrogen and progesterone to prepare the endometrium, knows that it is not needed because conception did not occur. If conception occurs, another hormone produced by the trophoblast signals the corpus luteum to produce estrogen and progesterone. This hormone, human chorionic gonadotropin (HCG), is the hormone that turns pregnancy tests positive. Without this hormone signal to the corpus luteum, the production of estrogen and progesterone ceases. The lack of these two hormones to nourish the endometrium causes the endometrium to shed, a phenomenon we call menses.

Since estrogen and progesterone counteract insulin, the action of insulin is weaker during the luteal phase. Since estrogen and progesterone are the highest during the last week of the cycle, this week requires the most insulin. In other words, it takes more insulin to keep the blood sugar normal even where there is no change in food intake.

June and Barbara: How does a woman go about adjusting her insulin to accommodate all of this?

Dr. Jovanovic: Once she begins to ovulate, a woman's hormone pattern should be fairly consistent and predictable, even though the hormone levels may vary slightly from month to month. By learning from one month's insulin requirement, you can make an informed decision about how much insulin to take next month. The first step is to discover when these hormone surges occur. Since you may not feel any different, the only sure way to tell is to watch the calendar and test your blood as soon as you get up every morning. You want to know the *fasting* blood-glucose level, so you should monitor your blood sugar before you eat breakfast.

When you know that this rise is occurring, you can slowly increase your insulin dosage, particularly in the overnight insulins, which are designed to have you in the normal range of blood sugar when you wake up. Since estrogen and progesterone are working against insulin throughout this five-day period, you need to have slightly more insulin circulating in your blood the entire time. This means that you require slightly more long-acting insulin (NPH, lente, or ultralente insulin), or, if you're using the insulin pump, more "basal" flow of regular insulin.

The insulin dosage should be raised *very gradually* (by perhaps 3 percent a day over a five-day period). This may not be enough to get your blood sugar level back to normal the first month, but at least you'll know where to start your dosage when the next month rolls around. As soon as you see the first stain of blood, immediately drop the insulin dose back to the original starting dosage, because the estrogen and progesterone levels have already dropped back to their normal baseline levels. It's important to decrease the insulin dosage at this time so that you don't have an episode of low blood sugar in the middle of the night. As always, you should consult your own physician before changing your insulin dosage.

June and Barbara: We hear a lot about premenstrual syndrome (PMS) these days. Could you define it and describe how it might particularly affect diabetic women?

Dr. Jovanovic: Premenstrual syndrome is a term that is used very loosely. Many women have some symptoms—bloating or increased water retention, menstrual cramps, acne, irritability, and depression—that are caused by high levels of progesterone in the blood. However, the term *premenstrual syndrome* applies only if these symptoms are incapacitating and interfere with work or home life.

If you have these symptoms and feel overwhelmed by them, your physician can give you a medication that can help to alleviate them after simple dietary changes have been made, such as avoiding salty foods, caffeine and chocolate. Antiprostaglandin agents are the best, for prostaglandin has been implicated as the major villain. Motrin is a very strong antiprostaglandin that I recommend to my patients. It's best to discuss these symptoms in conjunction with your premenstrual insulin requirements during the same visit to your physician.

You may also find that you can ease some of your moody feelings by keeping your blood sugar in good control. There has been scientific evidence to suggest that high blood sugar can contribute to depression, making premenstrual moodiness even worse. The anxiety you feel can raise your blood sugar even higher, so do try to keep your blood sugar in good control, even through these turbulent periods—because we all know those times are tough enough already!

Remember the credo "Know thyself." This is good advice in general, but it is particularly relevant to the woman with diabetes. By learning all you can about your own monthly cycle, you can gradually achieve and maintain that wholesome balance that keeps you feeling good.

June and Barbara: While on the subject of menstruation, we wrote in our first book, *Alice in Womanland*, about the pamphlets and women's magazine articles that "tell the newly pubertized girl who lies clutching a heating pad to her cramped innards, 'But, my dear, don't call it the *curse*. It's part of the *joy* of being a woman. It's a blessing and you should be happy to experience it, and, yes, *proud.*' " This struck us as so ludicrous that we took to referring to our monthly periods ironically as "the joy" or, with the delicacy of the French language, *"la joie."* At any rate, whether you regard cramps as pain or rapture, what causes them and how can they be avoided or gotten rid of?

Dr. Jovanovic: The chief cause of cramps is prostaglandins, which make the uterus contract. Any antiprostaglandin will work to prevent cramps, but high doses are needed, and many of these drugs have severe side effects at higher doses. Motrin (ibuprofen), which I mentioned before, has few side effects. Ordinary aspirin will work, too, but many times high dosages of aspirin are irritating to the stomach.

June and Barbara: Is there anything wrong with over-the-counter drugs like Midol?

Dr. Jovanovic: No, there's nothing wrong with them if they work. But for those who suffer from severe cramps my advice is to build up blood levels with drugs five days before the period is due. For example, take 400 mg of Motrin four times a day, at breakfast, lunch, dinner, and bedtime. This acts to contract the prostaglandins as they pour into the bloodstream *before* the cramps occur. It's much harder to stop cramps once they start.

June and Barbara: Are diabetic women more suscepti-ble to cramps than nondiabetic women?

Dr. Jovanovic: No. Poor diabetic control may prevent ovulation, and lack of ovulation is a reason for missed or scanty periods. But control doesn't seem to impact on the degree of pain of menstrual cramps.

Cramps are the normal pain response to a uterus clamping down to get rid of the old blood and tissue. Why the uterine muscle hurts so much when it contracts nobody knows. The Bible claims that labor pains are our punishment for partaking of the golden apple—but it doesn't seem fair that we feel this pain every month!

June and Barbara: As you might imagine, many young —and not quite so young—women have written us with questions about sex. Most of these questions can be boiled down to this: How does diabetes affect one's sex life?

Dr. Jovanovic: Sex is so simple to spell, yet so difficult to talk about. Perhaps it is our upbringing that pushes sex into the whispers of our conversations; perhaps it is our own insecurity that we are not good enough, not worthy enough, or not fortunate enough. But sex should be quite natural—after all, it is a bodily function. Dia-betic women have the same wonder about sex as nondia-betic women. The main difference is that if any small problem arises, many women have hidden fears that it is something about having diabetes that creates the prob-lem.

There are some situations that do impact on sex when a woman has diabetes. One example in particular comes to mind. If a woman thoroughly enjoys the sexual encounter, the sheer exercise of the experience may re-sult in a severe hypoglycemic episode. Thus, a woman needs to be prepared. She should adjust her insulin downward in anticipation of the evening, or, if the event happens on the spur of the moment, she should compensate by eating something afterward.

Libido is the word that describes our lust for sex. Psychological as well as hormonal factors control our libido. If a woman is sick, she certainly has no interest in sex. Likewise, if she is suffering from a severe vaginal infection, she would avoid a sexual encounter because of the fear of pain. High blood-glucose levels tend to be associated with increased problems with vaginitis, and it is therefore not surprising that so many diabetic women do not enjoy sex.

In addition, if the diabetes is out of control to a degree sufficient to cause delayed or missed periods, the normal cycling of hormones that increase libido doesn't occur. There are some diabetic women, on the other hand, who experience an *increase* in libido. These women have a syndrome of diabetes and polycystic ovarian disease that elevates the male hormone testosterone in their blood. Testosterone is the strongest libido-producing hormone.

Libido is also intimately associated with mood. If a woman is depressed, she cannot be easily seduced. In addition, if she does not feel sexy, she is not in the mood for sex. Unfortunately, being overweight is associated with Type II diabetes and also with not feeling sexy. It is true, too, that chronic hyperglycemia is associated with depression, and that's another reason why women with diabetes may not be interested in sex.

The best way to be sexy and enjoy sex, therefore, is to be happy, healthy, fit, and in good control of your blood-glucose levels.

June and Barbara: One complaint we've heard is that women are often neglected in studies of sex and diabetes, most of which are concerned with impotence in males.

Dr. Jovanovic: It's true that men have gotten most of the attention and there are several reasons for this. For one thing, women haven't complained loudly enough in the past. Perhaps the women's movement has taught us to be more assertive now. For another, when a man has no libido he cannot perform, for he will not be able to have an erection. When a woman has decreased libido, while it is true that she will not have adequate lubrication, she can still perform by using a bit of jelly. Finally, the first researchers in this field were men, and thus their interest was primarily in men. We women researchers have been guilty of investigating only female problems, too.

Now that women with diabetes have brought up this issue, a major laboratory at Columbia University has performed elegant studies to document a physiological etiology of decreased libido in certain women with diabetes.

Along with the information I gave you in the previous question, I can add that Dr. Judith Lorber, in her studies at Columbia, found that loss of libido can be caused by the following:

Out-of-control diabetes. Hyperglycemia can potentiate depression and a sense of being hopeless and helpless. Such feelings do not make one feel sexy. In addition, these blood-glucose levels take their toll on energy and vitality and can actually be a form of chronic illness, not to mention causing an increased susceptibility to infections.

Vaginal infections, specifically, moniliasis or candidiasis. These infections cause a terrible itching and increased pain on intercourse. The fear of pain can be a great turnoff to sex.

Neuropathy. Dr. Lorber has documented a form of diabetic neuropathy that affects the nerves to the geni-
tal area. This condition can prevent adequate lubrication as well as orgasmic climax. It is the same
condition present in the male diabetic person who
has impotence on an autonomic neuropathic basis.

June and Barbara: Since the one thing a diabetic woman
shouldn't have is an unplanned pregnancy before she
has achieved the good blood-sugar control that assures
a healthy baby, it stands to reason that she is going to
have to practice some form of birth control. Could you
give us a rundown of the various methods and recommend the ones that are best for diabetic women?

Dr. Jovanovic: There is now good news for the woman
with diabetes. If she does not have high blood pressure
or diabetic retinopathy, she may take low-dose birth-
control pills. Recent evidence shows that the hormonal
levels of these pills are so low that they are not associated
with an increase in the risk of thromboembolic disease.
In addition, the impact of these pills on insulin doses is
minimal. Even women who had gestational diabetes can
take this pill without fear of recurrent glucose intolerance.

However, despite the fact that they are an effective
means of birth control, there are some drawbacks to
these birth-control pills. For one thing, many women
experience spotting, which usually indicates that a
higher dose of hormone is needed—and higher doses of
hormones do impact on glucose and insulin requirements.

Unfortunately, the intrauterine device (IUD) is now
off the market, except for one with a progesterone addition. I say "unfortunately" because researchers finally
concluded that women with diabetes were not at a higher
risk of infections than nondiabetic women. (As you are

probably aware from all the publicity, IUDs were taken off the market due to mishaps that occurred in normal women without diabetes.)

Barrier methods such as the condom, diaphragm, and cervical sponge are only protective when they are in place. Certainly women with diabetes can use these, too, if they do so properly.

June and Barbara: What if a diabetic woman does not want to *ever* have children? Would a tubal ligation be hazardous?

Dr. Jovanovic: A tubal ligation is not a hazardous procedure and would not be hazardous in the case of a diabetic woman, but I would only recommend it when a woman is absolutely, *positively* certain that she does not want to have children.

June and Barbara: Do you ever recommend a vasectomy for the husband?

Dr. Jovanovic: Only when the husband requests it. I would not recommend it to a man on my own. I must admit that I feel confident to counsel a woman, but to extend that kind of advice to a husband—who is not my patient—is overstepping my bounds.

June and Barbara: Is there ever a time when you flat-out advise a woman not to have children?

Dr. Jovanovic: I do when a woman has diabetic kidney disease. Unfortunately, the statistics today say that after the onset of protein leakage into the urine from a damaged kidney, the patient is destined to be on dialysis within five years. Persons with diabetes do not usually do well on dialysis, and thus at least half of these persons are dead in another five years. With this stark information at hand, when a woman with diabetic kidney disease contemplates pregnancy I reassure her that her chances of having a healthy child are excellent with a program of blood-glucose normalization. However, I let her know that she may not live to see the child start kindergarten.

How does she feel about leaving her husband alone with a small child? Perhaps it is her way of making sure that her husband will not be alone, but will the burden be too great for him to bear? Only the woman can make this decision, not the physician. I can only state the facts in order to help her come to an educated decision.

June and Barbara: In answering the questions about sex, you mentioned vaginitis. We hear a lot about that from diabetic women. Are they more susceptible to it than nondiabetic women?

Dr. Jovanovic: Vaginitis is a normal female problem potentiated by diabetes. It's important to remember that with vaginitis a specific bacteriological *and* microscopic examination must be made. Vaginal discharges may look, feel, and smell the same, but the culprit bug could be any one or many from a large list. The only way to treat vaginitis, therefore, is to send some of the secretion to the laboratory for culture and to examine it under a microscope. There are four classifications of vaginal discharges:

1. *Normal.* No infection, just a large amount of secretions.
2. *Bacterial.* Example: hemophilus, gonorrhea, chlamydia.
3. *Parasites.* Example: *Trichomonas.*
4. *Yeast.* Example: *Candida.*

Each of the above organisms requires a different local care, and some necessitate that oral medication be taken. Some can actually be the cause of sterility. High blood-sugar levels can make these infections worse.

Without the appropriate therapy, the infection will never be cured. Therefore, unless the gynecologist takes a specimen for the laboratory and looks at it personally under the microscope, the cream prescribed may not be treating the infection at all.

June and Barbara: Since some vaginal discharges are normal and some are not, could you help us distinguish between the two?

Dr. Jovanovic: Normal vaginal discharge has different characteristics at different times. Early in the menstrual cycle it is mixed with the menstrual blood. From day five until day twelve, it is thick and very light yellow. It has a subtle, musky odor. On the day of ovulation, it becomes thin and watery, and then by day sixteen or so it is back to thick. It does not itch or stain.

A discharge usually associated with an infection is one that smells foul, has a brown or deep yellow color, may be as thick as cottage cheese, or itches and burns.

June and Barbara: One woman who has frequent vaginal infections wrote to ask if there is an approved way to collect the discharge and just bring it to the doctor to be cultured; this would save the time of having to go to the doctor with the complaint and then receive instructions on how to collect the sample. She also wondered if there are any home tests for vaginal discharges, just as there are now tests for blood sugar and for blood in the stool.

Dr. Jovanovic: There is no quick self-test. The discharge needs to be cultured for at least five kinds of bacteria, one kind of yeast, and one kind of parasite (*Trichomonas*). And these cultures need to be handled in a special way *immediately* after the specimen is taken, so this answers the first part of your question. The gynecologist can decide which culture to take after looking at the discharge under a microscope. Bacteria are small round circles, yeast looks like budding beads, and a trichomonad is a moving circle with a tail. Expertise takes a while to acquire, and a home test would thus be impossible.

June and Barbara: One woman asked us if there is any douche that is particularly recommended, or *not* recommended, for diabetic women.

Dr. Jovanovic: No, one douche over another is not necessarily better for women with diabetes. But the message is that if a woman has a vaginal infection manifested by discharge, odor, staining, or itching, she should seek medical advice. Vaginitis may adversely affect blood-sugar control, and poor blood-sugar control in turn adversely affects vaginitis. Specific medication for the problem is necessary. Over-the-counter douches will *not* cure the infection.

June and Barbara: Now let's explore some of the general problems and possibilities of Type I diabetes, those that pertain to Type I women of all ages.

The ideal way of achieving good control would seem to be to test your own blood sugar and adjust your own insulin dose accordingly, but that can be risky if you don't know what you're doing. How can you tell—and how can your *doctor* tell—if you're intelligent and sufficiently educated in diabetes to handle it?

Dr. Jovanovic: Your level of intelligence or formal education, the number of hours you've sat in diabetes classes, or even the number of books you've read on the subject are not the key issues in whether you're able to take on the responsibility of adjusting your own insulin. What is needed is a trial period. During this time, you don't actually change the doses of insulin you take but instead you record a minimum of a week's worth of blood-sugar tests, performed at least four times a day. In going over these records with your health-care professional you say which blood sugars you felt needed touching up and which insulin adjustments you would have made at the time.

In this way your health-care professional can learn if you're making knowledgeable decisions that indicate a true understanding of how the kinds of insulin you're taking work in your body under different life circumstances. If you make a wrong suggestion, you can be corrected and instructed in the insulin-dosage concept in which you've shown some confusion. All this learning takes place without the chance of your getting into trouble. It's rather like taking a course in investing in which you pretend to buy certain stocks and then see if they go up or down without actually risking real money.

You should not, of course, take over full command of your insulin therapy until you've shown proper judgment in all situations.

June and Barbara: June's been adjusting her own insulin for the last seven years, since she got a meter and was able to see accurately what her blood sugars were. She just kind of eased into a trial-and-error insulin-adjustment program. She did it without formal instruction, which wasn't available then, but it would have been a lot easier—and she probably would have made fewer mistakes—if she'd had a trial period such as the one you suggest. For the woman who's going to follow this trial-period plan, how long would you estimate it would take before she could confidently take over her insulin adjustment?

Dr. Jovanovic: Most surveys estimate that it takes about twenty hours of input from a health-care professional before you can expect to master all the skills necessary to take full command of the insulin-adjustment regime. Whether you're a high-school graduate or a Ph.D., it seems to take about the same amount of time.

If, after those twenty hours of intensive input, you still show errors of judgment in insulin dosage, then you shouldn't try to adjust your own insulin. To pick up the investment-class analogy again, if on paper you kept losing thousands and thousands of dollars, then you'd be more than foolish to start investing your hard-earned real money using the same bad judgment.

June and Barbara: It's too bad there isn't some kind of computer that you could feed all the information into and that would be programmed to tell you how to adjust your insulin.

Dr. Jovanovic: Oh, but there *is.* It's called the Pocket Doc, and it's a computer the size of a small calculator. The Pocket Doc contains in its memory all the necessary variables for deriving optimal insulin doses when those variables are placed into the mathematical formula specific to the individual's needs. The mathematical formula takes into account your body weight, the insulin-to-carbohydrate ratio (how much insulin it takes to cover ten grams of carbohydrate), and your metabolic status (e.g., growing child, pregnant woman, etc.).

Then all you have to do is put your premeal blood-sugar reading into the computer along with the carbohydrate content in grams of the meal you're planning to eat. The computer will then tell you the dose of insulin you need to cover this meal.

The Pocket Doc has in its memory a running total of the meal plan, average blood sugars, and times of day these blood-sugar levels occurred. Based on these data, the computer will adjust your insulin doses upward or downward, "learning" from one day to the next until it finally arrives at the perfect doses of insulin for you.

June and Barbara: June's already licking her chops over the idea of getting one of these, because even after all her years of insulin adjustment she still has some doubts and makes some errors. Are Pocket Docs readily available, and, if so, how much do they cost?

Dr. Jovanovic: As we write this, the Pocket Docs are not yet available—but they probably will be by the time this book is published. For information about the development of these computers anyone can write to me at the Sansum Medical Research Foundation, 2219 Bath St., Santa Barbara, CA 93105.

June and Barbara: People can also contact us at the Sugarfree Center, because we intend to have the Pocket Docs there the moment they're ready.

On to another question. We all prefer tight blood-sugar control, but aren't there some conditions, such as heart problems, when it's a good idea to have blood sugars a little on the high side? And if so, how high?

Dr. Jovanovic: I can think of two situations in which control needs to be a little looser: a child under the age of seven, or a person with heart disease.

Children under seven do not have the muscle coordination necessary to take full charge of their own diabetes. If a low blood sugar were coming on, they could not take responsibility to check and fix it. Recent psychological studies have shown a connection between severe childhood hypoglycemic episodes and decreased intelligence. This is the danger with tight control.

As I said before, the number of years a child has diabetes before puberty does not play a role in the subsequent development of complications. Therefore, to help the parents and child get a good night's sleep, a rule of thumb would be to give the child a large bedtime snack, even if this caused the blood sugar to be a bit high all night (180–240 mg/dl). As the child reaches puberty (at approximately eight years and up), every attempt should be made to tighten control, because at that point the clock starts ticking toward complications unless blood sugars are normalized.

Now, about those with heart disease: Hypoglycemia is associated with an outpouring of adrenaline. This hormone produces the energy of "fight or flight," which means that the pulse races and the blood pressure and blood sugar go up. If a person has a limited cardiac reserve because of poor blood flow from atherosclerotic coronary-artery disease, the hypoglycemia could lead to a heart attack. Although this event is unlikely, persons with diabetes and atherosclerotic heart disease should maintain blood-glucose levels of above 100 mg/dl.

June and Barbara: One of our major missions has always been to spread the word about the dangers of hyperglycemia and to teach diabetic women that high blood sugars can be avoided with the self-knowledge gained through blood-sugar self-testing. We were appalled by people who were willing to run around with blood sugars over 200 and even 300, risking frightening long-range complications.

Now, after years of preaching control of hyperglycemia, we're starting to find a new phenomenon. Some insulin-dependent diabetic people have received such a strong message about the dangers of high blood sugar that they've switched to the opposite extreme and are embracing constant low blood sugars as the preferred alternative to ever going over 100. They seem to have lost all fear of insulin shock.

The following anonymous letter from a young woman is just one of several we've received about the perils of insulin shock:

Have I got a low-blood-sugar story for you! After years (eleven, to be exact) of walking around (or rather dragging around) with extremely high blood sugars, I saw the light and began an intensive management routine of four injections and five to seven blood tests per day. (I was inspired to do this after reading the Peterson/Jovanovic book.) I had always been afraid of hypoglycemia, and I now realize it was because my former therapy involved taking only one whopping shot of long-range insulin (sixty units of NPH) every day. I had never had any dietary counseling and didn't practice any real consistency in meal and snack times. Consequently, the afternoon hypoglycemic "punch" packed by that large dose of NPH was disturbing and extremely uncomfortable. I had assumed that if I went on a multiple-injection program, my blood sugar would be even more precarious, and I'd have that horrible afternoon confusion all of the time.

Imagine my delight when, once I got real control, I discovered that I could function quite well with no symptoms at all, even when my glucose was in the 40–50 range. Cool! Neat!! Free sailing from now on. I then adopted the "lower-the-better" routine. I even tempted fate when exercising. Even though I had precalibrated my favorite remedy (five jelly beans = 30 mg rise in blood sugar), I hesitated to take it, for when I got home from exercising, wouldn't it be better to record a 60 in my diary rather than a 90?

One evening in early December, I got home from work feeling tense and knew I wanted to take a walk around one of Minneapolis's beautiful inner-city lakes (about three miles). The temperature was five degrees above zero, but being a native Minnesotan, I was prepared with adequate clothing. I took two fewer units than usual of regular insulin, ate my usual supper featuring 50 grams of carbohydrate, packed my jelly beans, and set out.

The jogging path where I usually walk is consistently heavily populated, so I had no qualms about going out by myself, even though it was dark. When I reached the lake, however, the path was slick with ice, and I decided to walk the perimeter on a sidewalk a few hundred feet away, on the edge of a residential section (dark and *un*populated).

I also realized it was a lot colder than I'd anticipated (with the wind chill, which I hadn't bothered to check, it was actually −45°). Probably due to the fact that I was using a lot of calories to keep warm, I began to feel light-headed after about twenty minutes of walking, yet I stubbornly refused to eat the sugar. After about twenty more minutes, I was barely able to think clearly, so I reached for the beans, only to find them frozen solid.

By that time, it was too late anyway, and I fell headfirst into a snowbank. It was simply luck that a passing pedestrian saw me tumble. If I had fallen when no one was around, I probably wouldn't have been discovered until the next morning, either dead as a doornail or severely frostbitten.

I am tempted to chuckle about this incident, for I feel humor is a very useful tool, but it's not all that funny. If fact, it is so embarrassing that I am declining to sign my name to this.

What would I suggest after this happened to me? To never exercise alone? Of course not. But be prepared, don't take chances, and keep in mind that one's life is more important than "perfect" numbers in one's blood-sugar diary.

Even if it had been light out and had not been during winter, I probably would not have carried my meter or strips with me. I justify this because it is difficult enough for me to interrupt my normal daily routine to make the tests, and I don't want to drag all that stuff around during my leisure time. But I was reasonably sure that hypoglycemia was setting in, and like a fool I persisted anyway.

Has this incident changed my way of thinking? Not really. I need to remind myself of this near-miss often and to also keep in mind that if I do overshoot with the sugar, I now have the tools to bring my blood glucose down to normal range with an extra squirt of regular.

Some things will no doubt take me a lifetime to figure out, but I would still advise anyone taking a single injection per day to give multiples a try. This system has afforded me more flexibility and dietary freedom than I ever thought possible, not to mention "euglycemia." (I love that term.)

P.S. I now carry the jelly beans in a pocket next to my body, where they stay close to body temperature.

This story—and others like it—put us in mind of one of James Thurber's *Fables for Our Time,* "The Bear Who Let It Alone."

Thurber described a hard-drinking bear who would reel home at night, knock down the lamps, ram his elbows through windows, and then collapse on the floor and fall asleep. His wife was distressed, and his children were very frightened.

Then, suddenly, the bear reformed and became a famous teetotaler. He told everybody who came to the house how strong and well he had become since he stopped drinking. To prove it, he would stand on his head and on his hands and turn cartwheels, knocking down the lamps and ramming his elbows through windows. Then, tired by his healthy exercise, he would lie down on the floor and go to sleep. His wife was distressed, and his children were very frightened.

Moral: YOU MIGHT AS WELL FALL FLAT ON YOUR FACE AS LEAN OVER TOO FAR BACKWARD.

It is admittedly difficult to walk the euglycemic tightrope of perfect control without toppling off from time to time. Is there *any* way you can be sure of never having a hypoglycemic reaction? June still has them on occasion. Are you, yourself, able to avoid them entirely?

Dr. Jovanovic: When a person has a blood-glucose level of 200–300 mg/dl all the time, she has plenty of room to fall—even as much as 100 points at a time. But when you keep your blood sugar in the recommended range of around 100 and if each unit of insulin can bring the blood glucose down 25 points, then an overcalculation of two units of insulin, or a matching undercalculation of twenty grams of carbohydrate, can result in bad hypoglycemia if the blood-glucose level falls much below 100 mg/dl. Sometimes a bit more exercise than usual can precipitate a hypoglycemic reaction.

Sure, I could prevent hypoglycemic reactions by *never* having a blood sugar below 200 mg/dl, but then I am at greater risk for complications of diabetes. The solution is to be prepared. Pocket food and desk-drawer juices are ever-present.

Even with all that, yes, I have been caught unaware when I was terribly distracted by a busy work schedule and have drifted into never-never land. Yes, it *is* embarrassing, but every time I make a blooper it makes me more determined to try harder to prevent these occurrences. In one case I passed out at a dinner party because the service was poor. (Ironically, this was a party at the National Diabetes Association Meeting, and fifty of the most prominent diabetologists in America seemed more prone to panic than to coming to my rescue!) Another time I was in an airplane so small that the hand luggage was put into the nose of the plane and I couldn't get to my food supply. I became so low I had a convulsion and ended up in the emergency room of a Detroit hospital.

I certainly don't like to admit my bloopers, but if I can learn from my mistakes to prevent another such episode in myself as well as in my patients, then it's worth retelling the experiences.

June and Barbara: We feel that it's vital for every insulin-taking diabetic to keep glucagon on hand. Glucagon is the hormone that can be injected just like insulin to revive an unconscious diabetic. How long can you safely keep glucagon?

Dr. Jovanovic: Glucagon is stable for up to five years in the form of a lyophilized (that is, freeze-dried) powder. Once the glucagon has been reconstituted in the special diluting liquid, it is stable for only one month in the syringe when it is refrigerated. I usually suggest that a patient have in the refrigerator at all times a syringe of glucagon that is current, labeled with the date that a new syringe must be made. Yes, it does seem a waste to keep putting fresh syringes into the fridge every month if they're not used, but I guarantee that no matter how savvy about diabetes friends or family members—especially, husbands of pregnant diabetic women—are, they are all toes in a crisis and cannot swiftly mix up the glucagon and succeed in injecting it. They tend to panic and can only manage to grab a ready-made syringe and find the strength to zap their beloveds. It is best, therefore, to indulge in the luxury of ready-made glucagon rather than keep it in the powdered state.

June and Barbara: There's a brand-new middle-ground possibility that we've just heard about—a small glucagon kit with a syringe preloaded with dilutant. All the person has to do is inject the dilutant into the vial of powder and draw it out again. Even a fairly panicked person could probably manage that.

Glucagon is manufactured by the Eli Lilly Company and is available only with a physician's prescription. This has always struck us as strange because insulin, which can cause death in the hands of the "insulin killers" you read about in the papers, is *not* a prescription item, whereas glucagon, which can rescue a person from the extremes of hypoglycemia, requires a prescription. We feel that the inconvenience of this keeps many diabetics from getting glucagon.

To turn to the other end of the blood-sugar scale, many women complain of frequently waking up with high blood sugars when they had been normal the night before. Some of them have been told that they have "Somogiied" in the night or that they've experienced the "dawn phenomenon." Could you explain what these two are?

Dr. Jovanovic: Somogii is a hypoglycemic episode that takes place around three in the morning. You sleep through it, and it is associated with the following:

1. having a bad dream
2. waking up with a low temperature
3. waking up with high blood sugar as a compensatory response to the low blood sugar
4. waking up with ketones in the urine from using fat breakdown to bring up the low blood sugar

Dr. Somogii was a Hungarian who described this phenomenon in 1956 and claimed it was due to an overdose of the morning NPH; his name was given to this syndrome. Technically, a low at 3 A.M. from bedtime NPH or regular cannot be called Somogii, although the wake-up high blood sugar is caused by the same compensatory mechanisms.

Since I try to be a purist, I use the word *bounce* to describe the phenomenon of a low followed three hours later by a high. When blood sugar is low, it signals adrenalin (epinephrine and norepinephrine), glucagon, growth hormone, and cortisol (in that order) to pour out and go to the liver and break down glycogen to produce sugar. The liver pours out sugar over the next three hours, and the result is usually a very high blood sugar.

Then there's what's known as the dawn phenomenon. The wake-up hormones, cortisol and growth hormone, rise with the sun. These hormones provide the trigger that gets us up to go in the morning. They are also anti-insulin in nature in that they make the action of insulin weaker. The blood sugar will rise if more insulin is not taken. This rise of the morning blood sugar between 3 and 9 A.M. is called the dawn phenomenon.

If a 3 A.M. low happens, the four stress hormones mentioned above will add to the two wake-up hormones to cause the blood sugar to bounce even higher.

Whether you feel your problem is Somogii or the dawn phenomenon, the strategy for avoiding high wake-up blood sugar is the same. You must prevent the 3:00 A.M. blood sugar from dropping below 70 mg/dl and you must have extra insulin available from 4:00 A.M. onward.

The ways to avoid dropping below 70 around 3:00 A.M. are to increase your bedtime snack or to decrease your evening long-acting insulin (NPH, lente or ultralente). For those on a pump, decrease your bedtime basal. To control the 4:00 A.M. rise, switch your before-dinner injection of long-acting insulin to a before-bedtime injection (this delays the peaking and may coincide better with your wake-up hormones). If on a pump, add more insulin to the basal rate after 4:00 A.M.

June and Barbara: Women, especially those who live alone, often fear having a reaction while they're asleep. Do you think the Sleep Sentry would be of help to them?

Dr. Jovanovic: The Sleep Sentry, a wristwatch-like device that measures two symptoms of hypoglycemia—a lowered skin temperature and perspiration on the skin—would be great except in the case of someone who does not sweat with hypoglycemia (80 percent of people with diabetes *do* sweat) or who sweats when she sleeps even when she's *not* having a hypoglycemic reaction (for example, during a menopausal hot flash).

Incidentally, the Sleep Sentry could be very good

for small children, or more importantly, for their *parents*, who could at last get a good night's sleep if they knew they would be warned if the child's blood sugar started plummeting. For *very* small children, the Sleep Sentry can be placed on the ankle rather than the wrist.

June and Barbara: Since it's often a battle to keep blood sugars normal, we get many questions asking what new therapies are available to help win that battle. Fortunately, there are more new treatments every day, including jet-injection therapy, the pump, and, still in the experimental phase, implanted insulin infusors.

Dr. Jovanovic: You mentioned that June is on jet therapy. That's one of the newer options for diabetic women. Perhaps you could tell of her experiences with jet injection and what it has done for her control.

June and Barbara: It's a long story, but we'll be glad to tell it. But then you must tell about your experiences with another of the new options, the pump.

Since June started on jet-injection therapy, she finds that if she's following her regular diet and exercise program, stress is almost the *only* thing that puts her blood sugar out of kilter. (See related question in Chapter 1.)

Jet injection has been around for quite a while. The first instrument, which was called the Hypospray, dates back to 1947. By 1962 jet injection was being used for smallpox vaccinations. With this method the substance being injected shoots in so fast—literally at the speed of a jet plane—that it becomes like a liquid needle and penetrates the skin almost painlessly. The "power pack" for jet injection is a series of springs inside the instrument. These springs are wound up prior to the pressing of the button that fires the injection off.

By the 1970s, what we know as the Medi-Jector had

been developed. However, it was not used for insulin injection until 1979, when the Derata Company was founded by a man who had an eleven-year-old diabetic son. This man adapted the Medi-Jector I for his son's insulin therapy.

Now there are two Medi-Jectors (the II and the LV), plus two other jet injectors, the Preci-Jet and the Vitajet. The prices range from $650 to $825. This is pretty steep, but reimbursement from insurance has been fairly good and is getting better. The prices of the injectors also tend to fluctuate, and by the time you read this some companies may have lowered their prices—or raised them.

As far as June was concerned, jet injectors were great for people with needle-phobia. Jets could well make them willing to take the two or three shots a day necessary for good therapy. But as for using one herself, she never even considered it. She didn't mind needles, and she felt that a jet injector would be both an unnecessary expense and too much trouble for her.

But because we always test everything we offer at the Sugarfree Center, June volunteered along with two of our other diabetic employees to take part in an FDA study of one of the new injectors.

As chance would have it, during the course of the study June had to have surgery to replace a joint in her hand. From bitter experiences in the past, June has learned always to get her doctor's approval to handle her own diabetes in the hospital. But because this occasion involved hand surgery, she wouldn't be able to measure or inject her insulin or take her blood sugars herself. This would have been a big problem without the jet injector. June trusts Barbara in most areas, including the taking of blood sugars, but she does *not* trust her when it comes to measuring and injecting her insulin; it's just too difficult for an inexperienced person to inject air into the insulin bottles, measure the insulin exactly, get the bubbles out of the syringe, and so on. With the jet injector, though, Barbara could handle the injections with ease and precision because the insulin is wound in by number of units and bubbles are no problem. What was even more remarkable in this case was that despite the stresses June was under because of the surgery, of being in the hospital, and of having alien hands administer the insulin, her blood sugars were absolutely normal during both the hospital stay and the recovery period.

At the end of the first half of the study, when June had to return the jet injector and go back on needles for the second half, June almost cried—well, at least she pouted a lot! As she sadly stated, "I didn't realize how much I hated needles until I got rid of them."

As soon as she got off the needle part of the study, June got her own jet injector, and something even more amazing happened. Her insulin requirements started going down, *and* her control improved. Figures 1 and 2 present two graphs that illustrate the difference between the two methods.

There are several reasons why we believe June's therapy was so improved with jet injection. As we mentioned previously, she takes a mixture of regular and ultralente insulins morning and night. When you inject with a syringe there is a tendency for the insulin to "depot," or pool, beneath the skin, changing the action of the different insulins. To avoid this June had been shooting her regular and ultralente separately. With her noontime regular shot, this added up to five injections a day. With the jet spray June could combine her doses again, since the insulin was immediately dispersed and there was no pooling (see Figure 3). The spray effect also speeded up and improved insulin absorption. June no

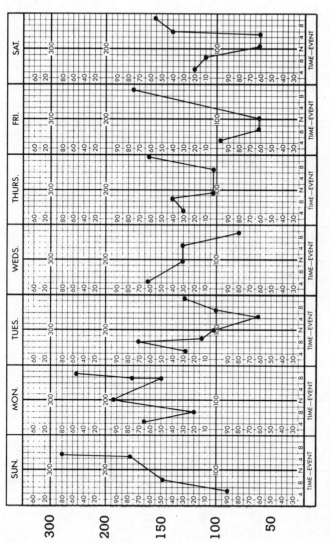

Fig. 1. Needle Therapy Week of March 10, 1984. Insulin dosage: 18 units plus supplements.

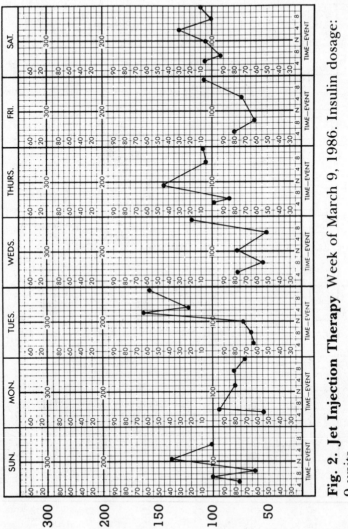

Fig. 2. Jet Injection Therapy Week of March 9, 1986. Insulin dosage: 9 units.

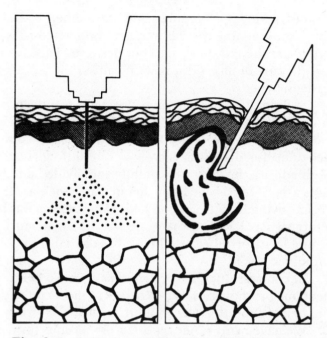

Fig. 3 Jet injection (left) and needle injection.

longer needed to get up early enough to take her insulin an hour before breakfast.

Another plus for June was that with jet injection, insulin's action is more predictable; it does what it's supposed to do when it's supposed to do it. The maddening frustration of doing everything right and still having things turn out wrong simply vanishes. June claims that this is an advance like no other.

As you can see from Figure 1, one of the most significant improvements is in her fasting (before breakfast) blood sugars. Prior to jet therapy June could never figure out why her fasting blood sugars varied so much. Was she Somogiing in the night? Was it the dawn phenomenon? Whatever it was, it is no more.

Since jet injection is so fast and easy, June later went

back to taking her regular and ultralente separately again, shooting the regular into her abdomen for fastest action and the ultralente into her derrière. This was the best therapy of all, and it is what caused the results recorded above.

Still another improvement for June has been psychological. As we related in *The Diabetic's Book,* when endocrinologist Robert Rood was the physician at a summer camp for diabetics, there was one little girl whose insulin dosage he increased slightly and divided into two shots a day. One day he found her in tears. She was afraid she was dying because, as she said, "My diabetes was bad before, when I had to take one shot. Now it must be getting lots worse because I have to take *two.* I'm going to die. I know it!"

In contrast, June's *decrease* in insulin gave her a tremendous psychological lift—"It says to me, 'You're getting better. You don't need all that insulin.' "

We have many other reports from jet-injector users who tell us that they now have improved control along with diminished insulin needs. But we're definitely not saying that jet injection is for everyone. Among the five diabetics at our Sugarfree Center, only June is on jet therapy. The others found that their therapy wasn't significantly improved by jet injection, probably because they didn't have an absorption problem to begin with. (June's doctor once told her that among the hardest patients to control are very slim older women, because such women often have problems with insulin absorption.)

One young diabetic woman on our staff has a life so crowded with activities—including settling into a new house, caring for her menagerie of exotic animals, attending classes for her nursing degree, and enjoying an active social life—that she feels it's faster and easier to use syringes. Jet injectors do demand a certain amount of care. Among other chores, you must disassemble them, boil them, and reassemble them every two weeks. There is, however, a promising new product called Vitaclean Germicidal, which is made by the company that makes Vitajet Injectors. We haven't tested this thoroughly enough to give it total approval, but it looks as though it may relieve the jet-injector user of the onorous cleaning chores described above. You simply draw up this fluid as you would insulin and shoot it into something like a folded paper towel, and the instrument is as cleaned and disinfected as if it had been disassembled and boiled. Other products of this sort from jet-injector manufacturers will probably be on the scene in the near future.

Many health professionals, most of whom don't have to inject themselves with a needle several times a day, have been dismissing the jet-spray injector as a gimmick or a crutch, and they claim that diabetics who resist sticking needles into their hides are "not accepting their disease." Our diabetic dietitian, Ron Brown, counters this dismissal, saying that it is "like saying that using an automatic finger-sticking device instead of jabbing yourself with a bare lancet is using a crutch or not accepting your diabetes."

Others claim that jet injectors are very dangerous. But *anything* can be dangerous if it is used incorrectly. Needles can be very dangerous if you stick them in your eye or ear or any place else they don't belong.

There is one negative factor about jet injection, however, and this is the high initial cost. The following table gives an idea of how long it takes to recover the costs of jets when compared to the costs of needles. The calculations are based on a person taking 30 units of insulin a day. Costs are shown for both two shots and three shots a day.

INITIAL COST
Medi-Jector LV: $725 (5-year warranty)
Preci-Jet: $625 (2-year warranty)
Vitajet: $650 (2-year warranty)

COST-RECOVERY PERIOD ON TWO SHOTS A DAY
Medi-Jector LV: 6 years   Preci-Jet: 4-6 years
Vitajet: 4.5 years

COST-RECOVERY PERIOD ON THREE SHOTS A DAY
Medi-Jector LV: 3.5 years   Preci-Jet: 2.8 years
Vitajet: 2.8 years

After the cost-recovery period, you are better off with jet therapy, since supplies for this cost only one-third to one-fourth as much as syringes. Also, you should take into consideration the possibility that your insulin dosage (and therefore your costs) may go down. Clearly, there is very little cost difference between syringes and jets over the long term.

As for insurance coverage, the jury's still out. Some companies pay; others do not. Jet injection is in about the same state as blood sugar self-testing was a few years ago. It takes a while for insurance companies to realize that an investment in something that can improve diabetes therapy is wise because if it prevents even one hospital visit, they're way ahead financially.

If you think you might be interested in jet therapy, we want to warn you that there's one thing it will not do: it will not allow you to ignore all the other aspects of your therapy. You cannot expect to stay in control simply because you're injecting your insulin in a different way. Jet injection is no substitute for your exercise, diet, and stress-reduction program. Nothing is! But for those for whom jet injection means the difference between a willingness to take multiple injections and a refusal to take more than one, as well as for those who have an absorption problem, jet therapy can mean the difference between good control and poor control.

Now, how about the pump? Since Dr. Jovanovic had that experience, let's let her tell it.

Dr. Jovanovic: Perhaps I should first describe a pump so that everyone will know exactly what we're talking about. An insulin-infusion pump is a battery-operated portable box that houses a syringe with at least a day's supply of insulin. The pump slowly pushes the plunger of the syringe so that insulin flows through a long tube that has a needle attached to the end. The needle is placed under the skin, usually in the abdomen, and is taped in place. The needle stays in place for one to three days and is then replaced by a new one.

The amount of insulin infused over the whole day (twenty-four hours) is called the basal rate. The basal rate is defined as that amount of insulin that keeps a Type I diabetic person normoglycemic (that is, with blood sugar always in the normal range) when she is not eating. When she wishes to eat, she simply pushes a button on the box to increase the dose of insulin to cover the meal. Only regular insulin is put into the syringe.

Usually the basal rate is calculated to be 0.3 times the weight of the person in kilograms. The overnight basal tends to be different from the daytime basal. From midnight until 4 A.M., the rate is usually 0.2 times the weight in kilograms, and from 4 A.M. to 10 A.M. it is usually 0.4 times the weight in kilograms. Once again, each person is different, so blood-glucose self-monitoring must be performed and the rate changed accordingly in order to derive the right basal rates.

The mealtime increased insulin need is about one unit of regular for every ten grams of carbohydrate in the meal to be eaten. This extra injection of regular (called the bolus) needs to be given far enough ahead of the meal so that the insulin and the food meet the bloodstream at the same moment.

Each person must derive her own lag time by starting a meal with a blood sugar of between 70 and 100 mg/dl, taking one unit of regular for every ten grams of carbohydrate in the meal to be eaten, and then checking blood sugar every fifteen minutes. When the blood sugar has dropped by 15 mg/dl, the meal can be eaten. The amount of time between the injection of the extra regular and the blood sugar's fall to 15 mg/dl is the lag time. This is the amount of time that must always elapse before you eat a meal.

June and Barbara: For which types of diabetics do you recommend the pump?

Dr. Jovanovic: Pumps are not for everyone. Many patients have stable blood-glucose levels on only one or two injections a day. A pump would not improve control. It would only make diabetes care more complicated.

In cases in which good glucose control can only be achieved with three or more injections a day, the pump can make the process of self-care a bit more convenient. A woman must earn her pump, however. If she is not willing to perform blood-glucose self-monitoring at least four times a day, she is not responsible enough to have an insulin pump. To keep the pump safe at least four blood-sugar tests a day are necessary.

June and Barbara: Now that we know what a pump is and how it works, tell us about your own experience with it.

Dr. Jovanovic: Six years ago I was very much antipump. I was bigoted enough to believe that control equal to that on an insulin pump could be achieved with numerous injections. Personally, however, I was having a terrible time on three injections a day of NPH and regular. Some days I would be high in the afternoon, and some days I would have a bad insulin reaction in the afternoon. Begrudgingly, I tried a pump.

Now, this was in the old days, when the pump was HUGE! The pump certainly smoothed out my afternoon dilemma, but I paid a dear price. I had to wear the "badge of courage." None of my clothes worked with a pump—certainly, none of my pretty clothes did. In addition, people thought of me as sick. "What is *that?*" they would ask. "Is it a life-support machine?"

And never mind the airport-security guards who ripped the pump off my belt to examine it better, pulling my needle out in the process!

Then there was the fear of sleeping alone. Of course all Type I diabetics have that fear to a certain extent, but wearing the pump exacerbated these fears. The reports of overnight hypoglycemia attacks had even *me* scared. Since I travel frequently, I am often alone in a hotel room, so I soon learned to pack provisions along with all my pump gear. Having to be dependent on an electrical outlet to keep my batteries charged also decreased my flexibility in traveling abroad.

In the total picture, I am not sure that the problems of wearing a huge pump didn't outweigh any advantages.

But then along came the "baby" pumps. These pumps could be easily hidden in even my prettiest clothes. The batteries now lasted a month, and I could get more flexibility in programming various basal rates. What a delight! My pump blues are gone—well, *almost* gone—now that I wear a small pump. I still have skin problems if I kept a needle in place even a teeny bit too long, and the tubing is still expensive. But I no longer feel like a freakish person in a crowd, carrying around my big black box.

June and Barbara: June talked on the telephone with a woman in Florida who has a small pump implanted in her chest. It pumps insulin in every hour. She can't alter the dosage, but she can take supplemental doses of regular insulin by needle.

This woman, whose name also happens to be June, has been diabetic for thirty years, since she was eleven years old. When she began blood-sugar monitoring and went on this infusion method, she was in such pain from neuropathy that she could not walk. It took two years and two weeks, but she now can walk for miles with no pain. To quote her, "This therapy has turned my life around and made me more of a normal person."

We found out that there are twenty people in the United States who are using this implanted pump on an experimental basis. This method is being perfected by Dr. Henry Buckwald of the University of Minnesota.

Dr. Jovanovic, could you give us some hints and hopes about other new therapies that are currently in the experimental phase?

Dr. Jovanovic: As the bioengineers are working on better pumps, the biochemists and scientists are working on transplantation of pancreatic tissue. If Type I diabetes is a disease of pancreatic fatigue, then the cure of the disease would be to replace the dead pancreas. Whole-pancreas transplantation is a very risky and difficult major operation. In addition, because the pancreas also makes digestive enzymes, if the pancreas is not hooked up properly the digestive enzymes could eat through the stomach and/or the gut. With all transplants, there is the problem of rejection. Our body knows that a transplanted pancreas does not belong to us, so it sends out attack weapons in the form of antibodies, which destroy the transplanted organ. Although the transplant may cure diabetes, the patient must take immunosuppression medicine to control the antibodies. These medicines have major side effects that can turn out to be worse than the complications of diabetes.

However, there is new hope on the horizon in the form of a transplanting of only the insulin-secreting cells. There is thus less foreign tissue to cause rejection, the digestive enzyme is not present, and the operation is technically a very easy one.

These cells do cause some rejection, and some form of immunosuppression must therefore be given. But researchers are working on treating the cells, rather than the patient, to prevent rejection.

June and Barbara: June (that is, "our" June!) is now on what is sometimes called the poor person's pump. This is not a pump at all but rather a different insulin plan. She first read about this in Dr. Richard K. Bernstein's book *Diabetes: The Glucograf Method for Normalizing Blood Sugar.* Before breakfast and dinner she takes ultralente, a long-acting (thirty-six hours), almost nonpeaking insulin that provides a basal dose similar to that of the real pump. She takes regular insulin before meals, which is rather like "bolusing" with the pump. This insulin plan has kept her in good control and has also reduced her incidents of hypoglycemia.

A diabetic supporting actress on a television series who took one shot of NPH a day often went into insulin shock if the taping went on past noon, as it frequently did. The whole crew would have to stop and revive her with juice or glucose tablets before they could go on. This was a great loss of time and money for the production company, and the actress began to worry that she would be dropped from the cast. However, when she started the poor person's pump plan, she found that she was able to continue working with no problem until the rest of the cast broke for lunch.

This is just one of the many insulin plans possible, based on your physical requirements and your lifestyle. *The Diabetes Self-Care Method* (Peterson and Jovanovic) has a wide selection of such plans that you and your physician can explore to learn which one can give you the best control and greatest flexibility.

We've mentioned insulin absorption as a problem that June experienced. How do you know whether you have this problem, and what can you do about it?

Dr. Jovanovic: If you inject the right amount of insulin to cover the meal you're going to eat and afterward your blood sugar rises for no apparent reason, then it's likely that the insulin did not absorb on schedule. My rule of thumb in that case is never to inject in that spot again. Absorption is slowed when the injection is made in a place where marks have been made by numerous insulin injections.

Absorption is *always* affected by the site of injection. Different areas on the body absorb insulin at different rates. Usually, the skin on the lower abdomen absorbs the fastest. There are several tricks you can perform to increase the absorption rate of insulin. After injecting the insulin, exercise the muscles where the injection was made. If you inject into the arm, do push-ups; if you inject in the leg, do knee-bends or jumping jacks. In addition, applying heat with a warm washcloth and/or vigorously rubbing the area of injection can increase absorption rates. Injection of insulin directly into muscle speeds up absorption by twenty minutes. I suggest using the calf muscle and then doing jumping jacks.

June and Barbara: Back when our dietitian, Ron Brown, was our first and only employee and before he had earned his R.D., he heard about the new purified-pork insulin. He marched out to a pharmacy and plunked down $18 apiece for two vials of NPH and regular. He explained, "I want to put only the best into my body. I don't care what it costs. I'm worth it."

We've come to feel that way about *all* diabetic people. They're worth it and should have only what we call "the champagnes of insulins"—purified pork and the even newer human insulin. Is this just a snobbish attitude we have, or *should* everyone be on these newer, purer insulins?

Dr. Jovanovic: I agree that someone starting out on insulin or someone who's on insulin only temporarily should only be put on purified-pork or human insulin so they won't develop antibodies. For someone who's been taking insulin for years though and who's been getting along fine on the so-called dirty insulins, I think it would be cruel to make them spend the extra three dollars or more per vial until it's definitely, absolutely proven to be detrimental to them.

June and Barbara: We have heard that the purified-pork and human insulins are less antigenic than the others and that as a result they are less likely to cause fat atrophy (lipoatrophy). The signs of such atrophy are the canyons and caverns that appear where insulin is repeatedly injected. Antibodies that your body produces in response to the beef/pork and beef insulins can gobble up fat cells at the injection site. This is not a pleasant state of affairs for anyone, but for young women who want to appear in shorts and bathing suits, it's particularly distressing.

We also heard from a young woman lawyer who's now happily back in bathing suits that if you shoot purified-pork or human insulin into the canyons and caverns, they may well fill in so you'll look as smooth as before. Have you found this to be the case, or do you think this woman's fat atrophy filled in for a different reason?

Dr. Jovanovic: Yes, the depressions caused by years of insulin injections with beef/pork insulin will eventually fill in if the highly purified insulins are injected first at the edges of the depressions. Then, as they fill in, the injections can be given closer and closer to the center of the depression.

June and Barbara: Another insulin prejudice we have is that we don't think anybody can have good therapy on only one shot of NPH a day. Is this true?

Dr. Jovanovic: Almost, but not quite. Diabetic women who still have some pancreatic function can get along on only one shot of NPH. The way they can check themselves for this is to see whether they always have normal fasting blood sugars. If they do, then this one-shot insulin therapy is all right for them. But no Type I diabetic without pancreatic function—and this is the vast majority —can possibly achieve optimum control with one shot of NPH a day.

June and Barbara: Here's a puzzling little ketone adventure based on June's personal experience. She was in Hawaii and got what was either food poisoning or the two-day flu. She treated it with Sugarfree 7-Up and chicken-noodle soup. During the sick period her blood sugars were all perfect—around 100—yet she had ketones. Can you explain why?

Dr. Jovanovic: Fat cells break down as a normal compensatory mechanism after all the sugar stores have been used up during fasting states. It takes about eighteen hours of fasting to use up the normal fuel stores of sugar, or glycogen, in the liver before fat begins to break down. Fat breakdown results in release of free fatty acids, which go to the liver and are metabolized there to ketone bodies. These ketones can be used by the brain as an alternate fuel source when sugar is used up.

June's illness, which resulted in almost no food intake but an increase in caloric expenditure due to the extra energy used when one has a fever, resulted in fat breakdown to provide her brain with necessary energy.

Fat will also break down spontaneously when the blood levels of insulin are absent or are very low. This is not a case of starvation ketosis, which happens to everyone, but rather of a person with Type I diabetes who has not taken sufficient insulin. Then there is a massive fat breakdown and a massive buildup of free fatty acids, which leads to ketoacidosis.

By the way, children and pregnant women need to fast for only six hours before they use up their liver glycogen and start to break down their fat stores. This is called accelerated starvation. Thus, in times of famine, saving the food for the pregnant women and the children was a very good idea.

June and Barbara: One of the unfortunate side effects of the women's movement is that women, especially young women, are drinking and smoking more. Let's take drinking first. Naturally, we know that drinking to excess is not even under consideration, but how about an occasional cocktail or glass of wine? What's the harm in that if there are no other contraindications?

Dr. Jovanovic: Alcohol seems to make insulin stronger, and it usually has its strongest potentiating effect four to six hours after drinking. If alcohol is consumed before bed, the potentiation may occur from 3 to 4 A.M., the very time when the overnight NPH or ultralente tends to lower the blood-sugar level. So I usually ask my diabetic women patients to restrict their evening drinking to one glass of wine and to make sure that their bedtime snack is large enough to prevent a 3 A.M. low.

If more than one glass of wine is drunk, then I ask the woman to take only one-half of her usual dose of NPH and still eat a large bedtime snack.

As you can see, it's easier not to drink at all rather than to second-guess the body's ability to handle the alcohol. Drinking is especially problematic when the drink also has a high sugar content. I usually dip a chemstrip into wine before drinking it to ensure that the wine is not overly sweet. By the way, I test diet sodas with a chemstrip if I think I may have been served the wrong drink. Regular Coca-Cola and 7-Up turn the stick to 800 mg/dl; diet drinks stay at 0.

June and Barbara: In every book we've written we've unleashed a tirade on the evils of smoking. We feel that no woman—in fact no animal, vegetable, or mineral—should ever smoke, under any circumstance. Do you agree?

Dr. Jovanovic: Definitely. Smoking is strongly linked to vascular problems, heart disease, and cancer, but for a diabetic person it has another terrifying consequence. At least 90 percent—and maybe closer to 99 percent—of diabetic people who need amputations are smokers. The good news is that five years on the wagon can reverse this risk.

June and Barbara: We once heard one of your colleagues, Dr. Douglas Muchmore of the Scripps Clinic, say, "I advise all of my patients who smoke to quit. For my diabetic patients, I *insist* on it."

Dr. Jovanovic: I agree.

June and Barbara: How about marijuana? We know the basic problems that it causes for everyone, but does it also cause special problems with diabetes control?

Dr. Jovanovic: The studies on what marijuana does to blood sugars are equivocal. Most studies say that if a patient does not eat uncontrollably, as with "the munchies," then marijuana has no effect on the blood sugar.

June and Barbara: How about other drugs, such as cocaine and heroin?

Dr. Jovanovic: No systematic studies on other illicit drugs have been performed, but I can't imagine why a diabetic woman would needlessly further complicate an already complicated life with drugs—not even on a one-time experimental basis.

June and Barbara: Of course there are other drugs, legal drugs, that are taken for physical conditions. How can these affect blood sugar?

Dr. Jovanovic: The following are drugs that don't mix well with diabetes or that may require readjustment of the insulin dosage:

1. *Hypertension medicines.* Diuretics raise the blood sugars. Beta blockers keep the body from releasing its own sugar in response to hypoglycemia.
2. *Arthritis medications.* Both steroids and nonsteroidal anti-inflammatory drugs raise the blood sugar.
3. *Seizure medications.* Phenhydantoin raises blood sugar.
4. *Cold remedies.* Unless they are sugar free, cough syrups raise blood sugar, as do decongestants containing neosynephrine and aphedrine.

June and Barbara: You mentioned steroids. When June was having a foot problem, the podiatrist injected cortisone, saying that it "probably would have no effect on her blood sugar." Wrong! Her blood sugars went so high that she had to increase her insulin by half. A young diabetic woman who worked at the Sugarfree Center was given cortisone for a knee problem, and she had to more than *double* her insulin.

I don't know if there are many diabetic women athletes out there who might be tempted to take steroids to build muscles the way some male athletes do, but if there are, would that have the same effect on their diabetes? Have you heard of any reports on this?

Dr. Jovanovic: I'm happy to say that I have never heard of a diabetic woman trying to build up muscles with steroids—and I hope I never do! If a woman did such a thing she would have to approximately double her usual dose of insulin to avoid high blood sugars. After two days of twice her normal dosage of insulin, she would find it would take another three days for the dosage to fall back to normal. For medical and ethical reasons, I would never prescribe steroids for any of my patients to use for improving their athletic capability. I would hope that most other physicians agree with me.

June and Barbara: Do you have any positive tips for women athletes?

Dr. Jovanovic: I would, of course, suggest that they take frequent blood sugars, since either hyperglycemia or hypoglycemia impairs athletic performance. Just as with Bill Carlson, the diabetic triathlete, the pump works well for some ballerinas—who are, in a very real sense, athletes—because they can disconnect it during practice periods and performances when they're exercising heavily.

June and Barbara: Speaking of exercise, since a diabetic shouldn't be sedentary, let's all stand up and stretch, do a little running in place, or even take a walk around the block before we move onward and upward into *le deuxième âge*.

Le Deuxième Âge

Calling this period in a woman's life the second age is particularly appropriate, because during these years a second is about all the time you have for yourself—if that! This period is also sometimes known as the "sandwich years," because you're often sandwiched between the demands and responsibilities of your young children and those of your aging parents, and everyone is trying to take a bite out of your time and energy.

The stresses of handling a career and/or marriage and/or motherhood, plus the built-in stresses of dealing with diabetes every day, can be almost overwhelming. You need to be aware of stress and learn how to handle it. (For books on stress reduction, see Appendix A.)

And yet, as stress expert Hans Selye says, "stress is the spice of life." These most stressful times are also very exciting times. If you can bring yourself to think of them as exciting rather than stressful, it will make them easier to accept and to cope with.

Since the excitement of giving birth is for most women a peak experience—and one that, until recent years, has been regarded as, if not impossible, then at least very risky and unadvisable for the woman diabetic —we'll devote the lioness's share of this chapter to pregnancy. Here we will explain the new discoveries and therapies that give a woman diabetic the same highly favorable prognosis as a nondiabetic woman for giving birth to a healthy baby.

June and Barbara: In one letter a woman gave voice to a problem that is probably common to all women embarking on a career or applying for a new job: "I still felt awkward about listing diabetes on a job application, especially when there is no particular place to list it. Do you feel it is better to mention it during a job interview, when you will have more time for a full explanation of how you control your diabetes? Sometimes the only question on a preliminary job application is 'Do you have any condition which will interfere with your ability to fulfill this job?' Would you ever mention diabetes in a résumé?"

Dr. Jovanovic: No. If I am qualified for a job, my diabetes should not be a reason to disqualify me. Unfortunately, an element of prejudice may creep into decisions about my qualifications if I mention my diabetes.

My diabetes is as private as my fibrocystic breast disease. Unless I am asked point-blank, I do not offer my health problems. Only such jobs as being a pilot or doing construction work on tall buildings would require that an applicant bring up diabetes.

June and Barbara: Here's one of those famous bad news, good news situations. The bad news is that you have diabetes, and the good news is that it may make for marital happiness.

At the Southern Illinois University School of Medicine, researchers were surprised and happy to learn that a disease as serious as diabetes could have a positive side. Despite the potential for conflict in the marriages of diabetics, the divorce and separation rate of a group of diabetic patients was relatively low. Only 21 percent had ended their marriages, compared to 46.6 percent among the general population.

Furthermore, a study reported in the *New York Times* found that "seriously ill women are more often than not blessed with loving husbands . . . marriage to such a woman means providing enormous support, and these marriages either founder or are very stable. . . . Marriages to sick women are different—there's more communication. . . . From poor men without jobs to bank presidents, these husbands have thought through their relationships carefully and are extremely loyal." This puts us in mind of Lee Iacocca, who, despite all the pressures of his high-powered work, was always tremendously caring and supportive of his diabetic wife.

Have you noticed this happy situation in your patients, and do you have any other insights as to why this is so?

Dr. Jovanovic: Perhaps the answer is that only special men choose wives with diabetes. It is as though they know we are not perfect but still find joy in the talents we have developed to compensate for our affliction.

June and Barbara: We all know that diabetes runs in families, so one of the first questions a diabetic woman has when contemplating pregnancy is whether or not she will pass diabetes on to her child.

Dr. Jovanovic: Yes, there is a chance that diabetes can be passed to the child, but the chances are less than 6 percent for someone with Type I diabetes. If you have Type II diabetes, the risk of passing it on to the child may rise to 25 percent. If you have gestational diabetes, it is possible that your daughters will also have gestational diabetes, and you yourself have a 60 percent chance of developing Type II diabetes.

Remember that babies are *not* born with diabetes. It usually occurs at eight to fourteen years of age. A rule of thumb is that if your child has inherited your genetic tendency to have diabetes and comes in contact with the "environmental trigger," then she or he will probably get diabetes at the same age that you did.

June and Barbara: On the subject of having children, one of our oldest friends coming to the Sugarfree Center is Sharon, a former diabetes nurse-educator who presented us with an interesting situation. She is a diabetic woman with many complications, including diabetic retinopathy, which requires laser treatments. Sharon and her husband, Glenn, agreed that because of her many health problems it would be better for them not to have any children. Fortunately, this decision has not caused them great personal anguish, since Glenn had never particularly wanted to have children anyway and it was thus not a major issue. However, they did have a problem with other people (as Sartre said, "Hell is other people"). On discovering that Sharon and Glenn have no children, many people seemed disturbed. When, after cooing something like, "Well, when are you and your husband going to start your little family?" they learned that the couple had no intention of having children, they were aghast.

Sharon became so tired of this that she started telling people that her doctor had absolutely forbidden her to become pregnant. This seemed to work, but Sharon said that she felt guilty laying the blame on the doctor when actually it was her and Glenn's decision (although the doctor did agree that their decision was a sound one). It was our opinion that Sharon should go ahead with what she was doing. We felt that it was nobody's business but hers and that the doctor probably wouldn't mind being implicated if he ever found out.

Dr. Jovanovic: I agree with your opinion that it's okay to ease the psychological burden of making a hard decision by sharing the decision making, or, in this case, the "blame," with the physician. I particularly remember one case of actual shared decision making that may illustrate this philosophy.

I was asked to advise a woman about whether or not she should have a therapeutic abortion. She had a glycosylated-hemoglobin level of 14 percent (more than twice the normal level), and she had been told that the risk of having a child with a birth defect was 20 to 30 percent. This also meant that she had a 70 to 80 percent chance of having a normal child. She was in terrible conflict and felt terribly guilty about wanting to abort.

I sensed this woman's ambivalence and distress over having to make this choice, yet I also sensed that she did not want to have a defective child if the risk was so high. Taking my cues from her, I took the responsibility and told her that if it were *my* decision I would abort, get myself into super diabetes control, and then start over to have a perfect baby. I therefore recommended that she undergo an abortion. Diabetic women usually have only one or two chances to bear children, and it would be a shame to invest time, energy, and money in a poor start.

This woman's depression lifted immediately. She felt relieved that she did not have to be the one to make such a decision. Her physician had told her what to do.

But, of course, I was listening to her soul when I advised her and recommended to her that she do what she didn't have the courage to do alone. Had her soul told me that she wanted this baby, no matter what, I would have told her to keep the child.

So you see, shared blame is okay.

June and Barbara: You mentioned earlier that it's not advisable for a woman on dialysis to get pregnant. What if she has a successful kidney transplant? Would that make it all right?

Dr. Jovanovic: Kidney transplantation has only been available for the last ten years to people with diabetes. When I was in medical school, persons with diabetes were not chosen for transplants but instead were left to die from kidney failure. This means that our experience with transplantation in those with diabetes is based on only a decade of experience.

During this decade only a handful of diabetic women with kidney transplants have had pregnancies. Although these women, their kidneys, and their babies did well, we will need more experience before I can say that all will be well after a kidney transplant. Ask me this question again in another ten years.

June and Barbara: In an article in the *New York Times,* "Having Children Despite Illness," the author, Jane Gross, explores the motivation behind the decision of chronically ill women to have children.

> Interviews with a half dozen chronically ill women and their doctors indicate that they are largely motivated by a desire to be normal, to test the body that has so often failed them, to be like everyone else.
>
> "When your pancreas doesn't work, there's the feeling that you're defective," said Donna Jornsay, a diabetic mother with a one-year-old daughter. "The desire to prove the rest of you works is absolutely compelling. Also, you're confronted with your own mortality so much sooner than other people, and the desire to see some piece of you live on is very strong."

Do you see these motivations for pregnancy among diabetic women, or do you find some other reasons that are more common?

Dr. Jovanovic: Personally, I think that diabetic women are overachievers because diabetes only happens to highly motivated, talented people! Your stories above are true, however.

June and Barbara: Dr. Janet Mitchell, the director of a high-risk pregnancy unit at Beth Israel hospital in Boston, has noticed that husbands tend to be more unsettled than their wives by hazardous pregnancies—"The mother puts the baby first, but he puts the mother first." Have you noticed this, too? If so, how do you think it affects the dynamics of the pregnancy?

Dr. Jovanovic: Yes, husbands do have trouble with a rocky course in pregnancy. They think it is their role to protect and care for their wives, and they feel impotent when the wife becomes sick or the baby is in jeopardy. It is also harder to have your beloved sick than to be sick yourself. These two emotions potentiate each other and can cause extreme anxiety.

One way to help alleviate the problem is to give the husband tasks and responsibilities, such as mixing and administering glucagon, if necessary, or waking up at 3 A.M. to help the wife do a middle-of-the-night blood-sugar check. During labor, husbands are also useful to perform the blood-sugar checks while the woman is busy doing her Lamaze breathing.

June and Barbara: The *New York Times* article on chronically ill women who decide to have children also pointed out that "other family members, especially children, are marked when a sick woman embarks on motherhood. Sometimes a mother is bedridden or limited in her physical activities. There may be tension in the house, which adults often try to hide. Always, children are asked to do more, tolerate more, understand more than those with healthy mothers."

Assuming that this is so, do you have any suggestions as to how the tensions can be diminished?

Dr. Jovanovic: Yes. Family therapy is needed for even the best-adjusted families. Often, there are many painful issues that are not discussed. Group therapy facilitates the verbalization of anger, pain, and rejection. A child may feel unloved because mommy eats first. The issue is a feeling of a lack of love, not an issue of the timing of dinner. Perhaps in other subconscious ways the mother has ignored the child's needs, a situation that would be easy to remedy if only she were aware of it.

The best way to have a child accept the mother's diabetes is to include the child on all blood-sugar checks and injections.

Whenever my kids fell and skinned a knee, instead of a bandage we would run for a blood-sugar check. After all, it was a free way to check the sugar, since they were bleeding anyway. My kids also know how to help me help myself whenever I am low. I need all the help I can get at those times. Let me share with you a letter from a patient of mine:

> Luke saved the day for me shortly after Andrew was born. My husband was working nights at the time, and Luke (who had just turned four at the time) woke up and came into my bed and found me barely conscious. My blood sugar was so low I couldn't talk to tell him what I needed. Luke got on the phone and dialed "0," told the operator I was sick and needed an ambulance. Thank God I taught him our address, which he gave to the operator. The operator kept him on the phone until the ambulance and police arrived and he let them in. Luke never panicked or cried, and stayed with me and the baby watching over us to make sure they didn't do anything wrong. He even showed them where I kept my meter and my husband's work number so he could come home. I was so proud— so happy I had talked to him of what to do in case of an emergency. For a while after that he was always watching what I ate, he was afraid of it happening again.

The only bad part of that experience was I couldn't tell them where the glucagon was, so they gave me tons of sugar in orange juice. When I was finally on my feet and tested my bood, it read "high" on my meter. But I was alive.

June and Barbara: Some couples fear pregnancy for a very realistic reason: they're afraid they won't be able to afford it. Concerning the expense of a diabetic woman's pregnancy, we remember the story in our *The Diabetic's Book* about a doctor who always calls in the bride's and the groom's parents. He asks, "Do you want to be grandparents? Okay, then, are you willing to help out with the medical expenses of the pregnancy?" The future grandparents always say yes, the doctor reported, and he added with a smile, "I always hold them to their word."

Amy, a diabetic employee of ours, had expenses that were doubtless much higher than most because of the relatively expensive hospital she went to and because of the thoroughness of the monitoring of the unborn child. She had two amniocenteses at $675 each, four ultrasounds at $275 each, two fetal echo checks at $300 each, and eight fetal nonstress tests at about $75 each. All this comes to a tidy $3,650. Also, the baby was in intensive care in the neonatal unit of the hospital for the first one or two days. One of our Sugarfree Center clients, who also recently gave birth, did not have amniocentesis at all because her physician didn't consider it necessary. She also paid much, much less for the other tests.

What is your assessment of the cost factor?

Dr. Jovanovic: The economics of a pregnancy complicated by diabetes have actually improved. Before home blood-glucose monitoring, a woman would be hospitalized for over half her pregnancy, so the usual hospital bill was around $40,000.

Now the major expense is fetal monitoring and testing. There is good news on the horizon, however, for as better tests become available the present protocols for multiple serial tests may become obsolete. These newer tests of fetal blood-vessel-flow parameters must be verified to correctly predict the fetus at risk before they become a part of clinical care. In the meantime, repetitive serial fetal monitoring is the only available tool we have to assure the obstetrician that the unborn child is safe inside.

June and Barbara: When our diabetic employee Amy was thinking about getting pregnant, one of her biggest worries was her age. At thirty-five, she knew the biological time clock might have ticked too long. Her concern was whether there is an age cutoff time at which it becomes inordinately risky for a diabetic woman to become pregnant.

Dr. Jovanovic: No, there isn't. But after the age of thirty-five *any* woman should have a test to ensure that mongolism does not occur. This is a test of the baby's chromosomes to see whether they are normal. All women over the age of thirty-five have a one-in-forty chance of having a genetically defective child. Whether or not they have diabetes does not increase this risk. Nor does it decrease the risk; diabetic women still suffer the ailments of normal women.

No matter how old a diabetic person is, she should complete the following four steps before conception:

1. consultation with an ophthalmologist to assure that eye status is stable
2. normal blood-pressure test and normal twenty-four-hour urine test for kidney function
3. normal gynecological examination
4. normal glycosylated-hemoglobin level

An okay on all of the above points gives permission to become pregnant.

June and Barbara: We would imagine that diabetes care differs somewhat while a woman is carrying her baby. What changes does a woman have to make in her self-therapy?

Dr. Jovanovic: She has to maintain the same good care as always, only more so. Pregnancy means an intensification of the self-care program. The goal is to maintain constant normal blood sugars. By normal I mean pre-meal blood sugars of 60–90 mg/dl and one-hour post-meal blood sugars of less than 140 mg/dl. The rule is that the better the mother's blood-sugar level, the better the baby. The only way to keep such strict control of blood-sugar levels is to check the level on a meter between five and ten times a day.

The total program consists of blood-sugar monitoring combined with at least three daily insulin injections and rigid meal planning (three meals and four snacks daily). With this kind of commitment to self-care, a diabetic woman can have a perfectly normal, healthy baby. Without it, the outcome of pregnancy can be much less than ideal. This is well verified by the fact that before 1922, when insulin became commercially available, no infant of a diabetic mother survived. Even after insulin came on the scene, up to 50 percent of pregnancies terminated in stillbirth. Today, a diabetic woman has the same chance of delivering a normal, healthy baby as a nondiabetic woman.

June and Barbara: One of our questioners had heard a diabetic woman must stay in bed during the last two months of pregnancy. Is this true?

Dr. Jovanovic: No. Diabetic women do not need to stay in bed. Bed rest is the preferred treatment for high blood pressure, preeclampsia (a toxic syndrome of pregnancy), and premature dilation of the cervix or premature labor. If a diabetic woman needs to stay in bed it is because she has one of these problems, *not* because of the diabetes itself.

June and Barbara: Many people have made the observation that diabetic women seem to have fat babies. Is this always the case?

Dr. Jovanovic: This is known as the "Big Bad Baby" syndrome and is totally preventable. In the past, many diabetic women did give birth to babies weighing more than twelve pounds. The dynamics of this phenomenon are simple.

At about the twenty-sixth week of pregnancy, the infant has a fully formed pancreas that is capable of secreting its own insulin. If the mother has abnormally high blood-glucose levels, the sugar crosses the placenta to the baby. The baby will work to lower the blood sugar by producing extra insulin in its pancreas, which causes the baby to grow bigger. Just as a person becomes fat by eating too much, the developing baby becomes fat when too much sugar is transported into its circulation.

On the other hand, if the blood-glucose level of the mother is normal, then the baby will not become "big and bad." All you have to do to cure the Big Bad Baby syndrome is to absolutely normalize blood-glucose levels during pregnancy.

June and Barbara: Another important question asked repeatedly is whether a diabetic woman has to have a cesarean instead of a normal delivery.

Dr. Jovanovic: No. A cesarean delivery is only indicated in specific cases. The indications of a c-section are:

1. too large a baby to deliver vaginally
2. malpresentation (breech)
3. uterine pathology
4. dysfunctional labor
5. repeat c-section

Problems two through five can happen to any woman, but problem one is usually a problem associated with diabetes. Good glucose control during pregnancy can help prevent the baby from becoming too fat. Thus, a woman can do something to decrease her chances of a c-section.

Previously, doctors delivered women with diabetes before the due date, when it was too early for vaginal delivery. Now, with improved glucose control and up-to-date fetal monitoring, the pregnancy can progress to the due date, and successful vaginal delivery is thus more likely.

June and Barbara: One diabetic woman who had her baby when she was in her thirties looked aghast when she was asked if she were going to have another. "Not on your life!" was her unequivocal reply. Although hers was not a complicated pregnancy and things went very smoothly, she couldn't take the thought of all those low blood sugars and all the constant monitoring. She was so tired of coping with her physiology that she didn't even want to nurse. It wasn't that she regretted in the slightest having her baby—he is the greatest joy of her and her husband's lives. But she had not the slightest desire to do it again. Her attitude was rather like the Japanese saying about climbing Mount Fuji: "He who doesn't do it once is a big fool. He who does it twice is a bigger fool."

Of course, this woman made these negative statements only a couple of months after the birth, and she may change her mind later. But do you generally find that once is enough for most diabetic women?

Dr. Jovanovic: Actually, I have found that most women have a letdown after the baby is born. They find that they are no longer special and no longer need extra attention; they are not involved in a miracle anymore. Somehow, being a nonpregnant diabetic woman does not hold the same glamour and require the same degree of care that a pregnant, high-risk diabetic woman has. During the ten years of our pregnancy and diabetes program in New York, three of my patients have had three children each, and twenty-two have had two. The remaining ninety-five have had only one baby each.

June and Barbara: We'd like to know if there is any optimal number of children a diabetic woman should have. Do the risks increase with each pregnancy?

Dr. Jovanovic: Diabetic women have the same chances as nondiabetic women. If a woman has a c-section for the first child, she will usually have c-sections for the rest of her children. Four are quite enough of that!

Also, in each subsequent gestational diabetic pregnancy the gestational diabetes gets worse.

June and Barbara: As an only child herself, Barbara feels they're not as bad as they're portrayed in legend and song. But do you find that many diabetic women do not like the idea of bringing up a spoiled, self-centered, lonely only child? And if so, do they sometimes opt for adoption after the first pregnancy?

Dr. Jovanovic: Sometimes, yes. Many of my patients have chosen to devote nine months of their lives to making a healthy baby, and they then adopt a second child to complete their family rather than stealing time from the first child to devote another nine months to intense self-care.

June and Barbara: The woman we mentioned who felt once was enough said that her husband is even more adamant than she—he absolutely refuses to go through it all again. Donna Jornsay, the diabetic woman who was quoted in the *New York Times* article "Having Children Despite Illness," made it sound as though her husband might echo those sentiments. She said he stopped sleeping during her ninth month of pregnancy because he was so afraid she would go into coma. The idea was so terrifying to him that he would wake her up as many as twenty times a night to make sure she was all right. She felt he was relieved when she was hospitalized because it was no longer his responsibility to keep her alive. Do you find this usual among husbands of diabetic women?

Dr. Jovanovic: Yes, if the husband does not know what to do to prevent the problem from occurring or to treat the problem if it does happen. Blood-glucose levels can be terrifying, but most of the time the insulin and/or the food pattern can be corrected to prevent unconsciousness due to extreme hypoglycemia.

June and Barbara: When Amy became pregnant, her doctor wanted her to keep her blood sugar between 80 and 120. This meant that, working this close to the line, she had to endure a number of rather dramatic hypoglycemic incidents. Once she almost passed out at work. This frightened us so much that we immediately called you to see if this could hurt the baby. You were very reassuring that it would cause no harm.

Dr. Jovanovic: It's true that transient hypoglycemia does not harm the unborn child. However, *hyper*glycemia (any blood sugar greater than 140) may harm the fetus; thus, for the sake of the fetus, it's worth running the risk of hypoglycemia to ensure that hyperglycemia does not happen.

Hypoglycemia is not, of course, pleasant for mothers-to-be and their anxious husbands, and there is no reason to put up with hypoglycemia if a change in insulin dose, diet, or exercise can fix the problem without causing hyperglycemia. Perhaps decreasing the dose of insulin per injection and increasing the number of injections will do the trick; perhaps adding between-meal snacks or changing to pump therapy will smooth out the glucose levels.

An important thing to remember is that the greatest risk to the fetus is a *swift change* in blood glucose. For instance, if a pregnant woman has blood sugar low enough to make her unconscious or unable to eat, her husband may panic and call an ambulance. The medics are trained to give large intravenous doses of sugar to any unconscious diabetic person, and blood glucose could thus go from 20 to 600 in minutes. While the level of 20 is probably not bothering the fetus, the swift change in glucose to severely hyperglycemic levels does harm the fetus.

Therefore, husbands should be trained in how to inject glucagon, just in case. We suggest that glucagon be prepared by the woman (powder dissolved and drawn up into a U100 insulin syringe) and kept in the refrigerator. The husband can be instructed to give half the syringe to his wife, wait ten minutes, and then give the other half, if necessary. This two-dose treatment minimizes the chance of overdosing initially. Once the woman is "with it," usually within fifteen minutes, she can check her blood sugar and eat food to induce the hypoglycemia to gently come back into the normal ranges.

June and Barbara: What do you recommend for treating hypoglycemia for your pregnant women?

Dr. Jovanovic: I recommend eight ounces of milk for a blood sugar documented to be less than 70 and associated with hypoglycemia symptoms. (A 60 may be normal if it's *stable,* but it may have been caught only while a woman was on her way down to zero.) Recheck the blood sugar in fifteen minutes and drink another glass of milk if necessary. Recheck again in fifteen minutes, and if the level is less than 70 drink a third glass of milk and eat a slice of bread. For minor hypoglycemia, most women do not require the third glass of milk.

If a woman is unresponsive or is unable to eat, then glucagon must be subcutaneously injected.

June and Barbara: Since the recommended blood-sugar levels for a pregnant diabetic woman are lower than for the general diabetic population, could you give us some guidelines?

Dr. Jovanovic: Yes. They are:

   Prebreakfast (fasting) goal: 55–70 mg/dl
   Prelunch goal: 55–70 mg/dl
   One hour after each meal: below 140 mg/dl
   Average blood sugar of all the premeals and all the
      postmeals (six per day) should be 80–85 mg/dl.

June and Barbara: Since these numbers differ from the standard normal range, should a pregnant woman's hemoglobin A_1C (the every-three-months monitor of blood glucose levels) be different, too?

Dr. Jovanovic: Yes, because pregnancy demands that the mean blood glucose be lower than for nonpregnant persons. Therefore, the "normal range" for most lab glycosylated-hemoglobin levels cannot be used to determine whether a pregnant woman is in good control. The ideal lab would be one that also has pregnancy norms. In addition, A_1C is affected by temperature, humidity, and technical expertise. Thus, the test can vary from month to month with the weather and the changeover of technical staff. The easiest way to use a local lab for the A_1C is to send the blood to the lab with a normal control. The best control would be a pregnant woman without diabetes who is in the same week of gestation. Short of such an ideal control, a fit, lean, athletic husband will do. (Athletes tend to have lower mean blood-glucose levels than nonathletes.) I then demand that the pregnant diabetic woman's HbA_1C be *lower* than her husband's before I would deem her to be in good control.

June and Barbara: Some women use an insulin-infusion pump during pregnancy. Is this recommended?

Dr. Jovanovic: Not necessarily. Pumps create special problems during pregnancy. Since there are no subcutaneous stores of insulin when a woman is on a pump, if the needle slips for more than four hours she can go into ketoacidosis. In addition, because of the change in skin sweat and temperature, it is easier to develop an infection at the needle site. Infection necessitates antibiotics and usually causes the blood glucose to rise, two situations that are definitely not wanted during pregnancy.

It is therefore not recommended that a woman be on a pump during pregnancy, but it is certainly worse to be in poor glucose control during pregnancy. Pregnancy is a special time during which permission is automatically granted to eat special foods, eat when no one else eats, test blood sugars frequently, sleep sufficiently, and so on. It is not a selfish act to spend time caring for yourself, for you are also caring for your unborn child.

Thus, it is somehow easier to take the time for three

injections and five to seven blood-glucose tests a day. The nonpregnant diabetic does not have this luxury in real life; the pregnant woman needs all the help she can get to make diabetes self-care easier. Therefore, I would never prescribe a pump for her. She can do equally as well on multiple injections. However, for the woman who is *planning* a pregnancy, I would prescribe the pump to help her get her act in order before pregnancy. Then when she gets pregnant she can stay on the pump, but must be fastidious about her needle site.

June and Barbara: Is it okay for a diabetic woman to breast-feed her baby, and, if so, are there any special precautions she should take?

Dr. Jovanovic: I firmly believe that if a woman with diabetes keeps her blood-glucose levels normal before and throughout pregnancy, she can have a normal infant. Why, then, should there be any reason not to breast-feed?

Before I began to advocate breast-feeding for my diabetic women patients, however, I wanted to be sure that it would be best for the baby. So we set up an experiment to look at the relationship of maternal blood glucose and insulin to milk glucose and insulin. We learned that the higher the mother's blood sugar, the sweeter the milk. In addition, insulin comes into the milk freely. We do not know the implications for the baby of drinking sugar-laden milk with regard to taste and preference and/or subsequent obesity and eating disorders. We do know that the insulin will not hurt the infant. (If insulin could be put into a glass of milk to make it work, none of us would inject it!) Therefore, the rule of thumb for assuring the most normal nutrition for the baby is that women should keep themselves in the best possible control.

We have learned that women must adjust their insulin dosages frequently while they are breast-feeding, because as the baby grows more sugar is siphoned to it. Usually, the increased food intake during the day compensates for this, but when the baby eats at 11 P.M. and 3 A.M., the next result is that the bedtime insulins must be cut way back. In fact, many women skip the bedtime dose of NPH insulin altogether. The other option is to overeat before bed to prevent a hypoglycemic reaction. However, most postpartum women are desperate to lose weight, and forcing themselves to eat at bedtime is therefore depressing.

June and Barbara: One diabetic mother wrote of a worry that must be common to all diabetic mothers of small children:

> One major problem I encountered as a diabetic mother was the possibility of having a severe insulin reaction when I was home alone with my baby and young children. I had no relatives living nearby, and for a while no close neighbors, as we lived in the country.
> To have someone check on me meant letting someone know where I was at all times. If they phoned while I was changing a diaper, out in the garden, or in town on errands, it would be a false alarm. If we arranged a preset time to call, what about all the hours in between when an insulin reaction could occur? My ultimate solution was to keep my blood sugars high at all times—this was in the days before home blood-sugar monitors. My husband was away a fair amount of the time on overnight business trips, which didn't help, either. My doctors told me I was damaging my health, but no doctor ever came up with a better solution.

Dr. Jovanovic: As she mentioned in passing, the blood-glucose monitoring that is now possible diminishes the problem. It doesn't mean, however, that low blood-sugar incidents can't happen to a diabetic mother.

One way she can avoid these is by realizing the times of potential hypoglycemia danger, based on when her insulin peaks and will drive down her blood sugar. For example, if she is on a program of NPH and regular insulin, blood-sugar tests *must* be performed two and a half hours after regular is injected and eight hours after NPH is injected. *Any* blood sugar less than 100 should be treated with milk until the blood sugar is greater than 100.

June and Barbara: Since youth is so revered in this country, many diabetic (and nondiabetic!) women find moving into the troisième age a depressing stage in life. We hope to be able to prove to you that it ain't necessarily so.

Le Troisième Âge

According to Browning, this is the "best is yet to be" time, "the last of life, for which the first was made." For a woman it can truly turn out to be the best time of all. Family responsibilities are diminished, and she can begin to think of herself—her health, her interests, and her career goals.

June has found that in this third age she's happier, more productive (often working 9–10-hour days and 7-day weeks when necessary), and having more exciting and positive experiences than ever before in her life. After careers as a writer and a college librarian, she's now able to devote all of her time and energy to diabetes education. And at age sixty-four she has seen the Sugarfree Center join with a large health network in order to make her and Barbara's longtime dream of having centers all over the country come true. She's eagerly looking forward to working hard to bring that about.

She's also not letting down in the sports and exercise area. After about ten years of being off skis because of other demands on her time, she's made plans to take up downhill skiing again the winter of this writing. She hasn't given up her other sports activities, either—she remains an enthusiastic biker despite having suffered a broken arm resulting from a skid and fall on rain-slick railroad tracks, and she's still an enthusiastic walker despite foot surgery for a couple of neuromas.

Many women diabetics her age are doing as much or more. But, alas, the majority of diabetics in the *troisième âge* are not. We see women every day who seem to have given up on life and on themselves. One day June answered the phone when a woman who had a meter appointment called in to say she couldn't make it. She offered as explanation the fact that she was sixty-five years old.

"So what?" thought June. "What does being sixty-five have to do with not keeping appointments?"

We've also noticed that a sadly large number of third-age women approach everything new with negative expectations. This is particularly true when it comes to learning how to use a blood-sugar meter. These meters are easier than ever to use, having been carefully designed so that a person of normal intelligence and dexterity can operate them with no difficulty. Yet these women approach the meters with fear and trembling, and they often come right out and say, "This is too much for me" or "I just can't handle mechanical things." Even if they don't say it, it's written all over their faces. And you know what? It turns out that these women *can't* work the meters. They can have lesson after lesson and explanation after explanation, and they still don't get it. Why? *Because they're certain they're not going to.* That negative certainty is like a lead shield dropping down and blocking all learning.

One of the participants in the Iron Man triathlon (participants swim 2.4 miles, bicycle 112 miles, and run 26 miles—all in one day!) recently said that the moment you start thinking you can't do it, it's all over. The negative thoughts will beat you every time. On the other hand, if you say over and over, like the little engine that could, "I think I can! I think I can!" then the battle's more than half won.

The other half of the battle involves taking the time to learn to do it right. In his book *The Road Less Traveled,* M. Scott Peck writes, "I and anyone who is not mentally defective can solve any problem if we are willing to take the time. . . . Many people simply do not take the time to solve problems."

Sitting down calmly and taking the time to really understand how to use a meter or any other product or piece of equipment associated with your diabetes care will pay tremendous dividends, and not just in improved diabetes control. A more important dividend is that you will learn, as Dr. Peck believes, that most of life's mechanical, intellectual, social, and spiritual problems are solvable if you are just willing both to take the time and to make the necessary changes.

Question: How many psychologists does it take to change a lightbulb?

Answer: Only one, but it can take a very long time, and the lightbulb has to really *want* to change.

It's even harder to change a person than a lightbulb —especially if that person has become somewhat set in her ways over the years. When you come right down to it, people can't be changed. They have to change themselves. But change they must, because changing is the key to survival and happiness.

This is particularly true for diabetic people, who, especially at first, have to make a huge number of changes. But there are rewards for your efforts: the reward of improved health and appearance and, best of all, the reward of becoming a person who is capable of making changes in all areas of life—in other words, a winner.

This resiliency is also a hallmark of youth. A *première âge* person who cannot make changes is an old person, but a person in the *troisième âge* who can make changes is young, whatever her birth certificate may say. So if you get your diabetes later in life, as many Type II diabetics do, you can regard it and the changes it causes you to make as rejuvenating forces.

"Great," you may say, "I have this diabetes and I need to make changes, and I know that if I do it will make a lot of big, positive differences in my life. But how do I *motivate* myself to make these changes?"

Motivation. Aye, there's the rub. It would be hard to count the number of sessions we've attended at diabetes conferences that deal with motivation and how diabetes health professionals can motivate their patients to start doing all the things they need to do.

After a great deal of thought in the matter, we've come to this conclusion:

DOWN WITH MOTIVATION!

We hear it almost every day: "(Heavy sigh) I just can't get myself motivated to . . . (lose weight, exercise every day, start testing my blood sugar, etc.)."

We have news for you. Motivation is not going to strike you like lightning. And motivation is not something that someone else—nurse, doctor, family member, friend—can bestow or force upon you. The whole idea of motivation is a trap. Just get in there and take the first step to lose weight, exercise, test your blood sugar, or whatever. Do it *without* motivation. And then, guess what? After you start actually doing whatever it is, *that's* when motivation comes and makes it easier for you to keep on doing it. We had one overweight woman at the center whom we were encouraging to start exercising. So we made a deal with her: she was to walk around the block every day for a week and then come back and tell us how it felt.

She didn't want to, and she groaned a lot, but she agreed to do it. A week later she came in and admitted that while she had hated doing it the first time, it had gotten a tiny bit better every day, until by the end of the week it wasn't bad at all. Since then she's gradually increased her daily walk to two miles, and she has her husband out walking with her. Now they're so motivated to keep it up that they seldom miss a day.

Motivation is like happiness—it's a by-product. When you're actively engaged in Doing Something, motivation sneaks up and zaps you when you least expect it. As Harvard psychologist Jerome Bruner says, "You're more likely to act yourself into feeling than feel yourself into action." So act! Read what Dr. Jovanovic tells you to do as a Type II diabetic, then leap up and do it!

June and Barbara: Diana Guthrie, an eminent diabetes nurse-educator at the Kansas Regional Medical Center in Wichita, once told us that the diabetics who most often come into the hospital with serious problems are Type IIs who have been ignoring their conditions. What advice do you have for these people, and what recommendations can you give for their preventive care?

Dr. Jovanovic: High blood glucose is associated with an increased risk of heart disease and stroke. In fact, even people with borderline glucose intolerance (high blood sugars but not high enough to meet the definition of diabetes) have an increased risk. Therefore, as health-care professionals interested in preventive medicine, we should lower the blood-glucose level back down toward normal.

There are several risk factors that potentiate the risk of heart attack and stroke:

1. hyperglycemia
2. hypertension
3. smoking
4. sedentary lifestyle
5. being male
6. aging
7. high uric acid (gout)

Although obesity carries with it a higher risk of sedentary life, high blood glucose, and diabetes, a fat person who has normal blood pressure and normal blood sugar and who leads an active life is not at risk. Thus, obesity is not a risk factor all by itself. Therefore, although I push diet as the mainstay of therapy for Type II diabetic women, I would not be a good physician if I gave up on the patient if she could not lose weight. I would try to bring the blood-glucose level down with pills and/or insulin if necessary and vigorously treat the blood pressure, start the patient on an exercise program, treat the gout (hyperuricemia), and be vehement about not smoking.

I ran the diabetes clinic for seven years at the New York Hospital. Of the 1000 patients who registered in that clinic during that time, 85 percent were obese, Type II diabetic women. I learned a lot from these women. Basically, they educated me on how to understand them.

Many of these women had had a lifelong problem with obesity. How could I reverse a lifetime of poor eating habits in one clinic visit? Clearly, a busy physician is not the right person to implement behavior modification. But I could direct the patient to a better support system—a dietitian who would translate my diet prescription into a meal plan, a diabetes educator to teach foot care and sick-day rules and reinforce blood-glucose testing techniques, an exercise program exclusively for fat women so they could feel comfortable wearing leotards, and a group therapy directed toward the chronic eating disorder. My role as the physician then became the coordinator and monitor of success. If my plan failed, then I could shift gears and begin again.

Yes, my patients gained weight in my weight-loss programs. But I improved the average glycosylated hemoglobin in our clinic by two percentage points.

I guess that I have only one standard of care. Since Type II diabetic women are older, I view each Type II woman as though she were my mother. "If this were my mother," I found myself saying, "then I would make sure that her blood-glucose levels were below the levels of risk for heart attack and stroke." The safe zone appears to be a fasting blood glucose of below 110 mg/dl and postprandial levels below 165 mg/dl. If I cannot help a patient to achieve this degree of control, I send her to a doctor who may have a different approach, one that is more effective for this patient, for I am not helping her as long as her glucose levels are in the risk zone.

Blood-glucose self-monitoring is a beautiful way to assess dietary management. If the meal plan is perfect, the postmeal glucose level should be below 165 mg/dl. If a patient measures her blood glucose one hour after the meal and finds her blood glucose to be above 165 mg/dl, we can then discuss what foods in that meal she did not tolerate. Was it the ketchup, because I forgot to teach her that ketchup has sugar? Was it the soup with hidden items that are not easily accounted for? Talking about the blood glucose takes the emphasis off the scale. Many of my patients would rather skip a visit than step on a scale. So I do not weigh my patients. Why should I, if obesity alone is not harmful?

June and Barbara: You mentioned bringing down blood-glucose levels of Type II women with pills that lower blood sugar if these women can't get into control with diet. Could you explain the use of these pills? Many people have the false impression that these are insulin pills. When June was diagnosed as having diabetes at the age of forty-five, she was considered a Type II and was allowed to try three of the pills—Orinase, Tolinase, and Diabinese—but they did not lower her blood sugar enough to prevent her from having to go onto insulin.

Dr. Jovanovic: Those three pills belong to the sulfonylurea family of drugs. The second generation of sulfonylurea compounds has recently been introduced in this country in the form of glipizide and glyburide. These two agents do not cause salt and water retention, as Diabinese did, and they can be given in very small doses. The small dose is an advantage because the side effect of abnormal heart rhythm is also less. These new agents can be given in one-hundredth of the dose of the first-generation pills. It is easy to outeat these pills, however, and therefore putting a patient on such a pill does not give her permission to stop her diet.

A new idea being tried is the use of pills in combination with insulin. It has recently been reported that when bedtime NPH insulin is used to lower the following morning's wake-up blood-glucose level, the pills are effective for daytime control. The high fasting blood glucose carries with it insulin resistance, so if NPH can lower the fasting, daytime control becomes easier.

June and Barbara: Once a Type II woman has been taught the strategy for controlling her diabetes, how can you make it work?

Dr. Jovanovic: Honesty and trust between patient and physician is what makes it work. The woman must tell me if what I have asked her to do is impossible. Then, and only then, can I tailor the plan to be right for her.

June and Barbara: When we attended a diabetes scientific update seminar we heard a doctor speak on a study he had done on the oral hypoglycemic agent Orinase. This study was done with turkeys. The doctor explained that he had a flock of 10,000 turkeys and that he had given each turkey one Orinase tablet morning and evening for six months.

At this point in the lecture one of the physicians in the audience raised his hand and said, "Excuse me, doctor, I don't want to interrupt your train of thought, but I have to ask you how you managed to get 10,000 turkeys to take an Orinase tablet every morning and evening."

"It was easy," replied the lecturer. "I told them that if they didn't take it, I'd put them on insulin."

But seriously, this story points up the great truth that everybody has a dread of going onto insulin. That's why a typical question we get goes like this: "I have Type II diabetes, and I'm scared that my doctor will put me on insulin if my control doesn't improve. What can I do to stay off insulin? I've lost some weight on his advice, but I admit that I'm still way too heavy."

Dr. Jovanovic: As many as 50 percent of all overweight Type II diabetics can control their diabetes by restricting calories and carbohydrates and eating more fiber. Not more than 40 percent of the diet should be carbohydrates. By getting your weight down by at least 20 percent you will most likely be able to control your diabetes without the use of insulin.

The reasoning behind this recommendation is that your pancreas probably *does* produce enough insulin, but your body resists the insulin. Losing weight and eating less will increase your sensitivity to insulin and improve your blood-sugar levels. The fiber in your diet will help lower your blood sugar by slowing down the absorption of glucose in the intestines. The oral hypoglycemic drugs may also help increase your sensitivity to your own insulin and prevent the need for additional injected insulin.

You can be the deciding factor in whether your doctor must prescribe pills or insulin. The goal is to normalize your blood sugar. If you can do this by following the correct diet and adding exercise to your daily program, your reward will be to stay healthy without the use of insulin injections.

June and Barbara: We've had letters from older Type I women who, after many years of diabetes, suddenly find that they no longer receive the usual signals that they have low blood sugar. One moment they are conscious, and the next moment they are unconscious. After a couple of experiences like this they are terrified and naturally want an explanation for this phenomenon. We usually advise them to test their blood sugar more frequently so that they won't get caught unaware.

Dr. Jovanovic: As I've said, menopause decreases the insulin requirement, and menopausal women are thus more predisposed to low blood glucose. Menopause does not decrease signals, but it occurs at a time when most Type I women have had at least twenty years of diabetes. Thus, the neuropathy of diabetes is what decreases the signals.

June and Barbara: The menopause is another significant life event for a woman and one about which we've received many questions, on both the physiological and the psychological aspects. Let's start with the physiology of menopause and how it can affect diabetes.

Dr. Jovanovic: The word *menopause* comes from the Greek: *men* means "month," and *pause* means "cessation"—thus, "permanent cessation of the monthly cycle."

With this cessation of the monthly cycle, the hormones necessary to maintain this cycle deteriorate. Specifically, the female hormones estrogen and progesterone diminish. Both of these hormones counteract the action of insulin; thus, as their levels diminish in the bloodstream, insulin's action increases. The insulin requirement will drop as the menses become fewer and farther apart. If the insulin doses are not decreased, hypoglycemia results. A drop of approximately 10 to 20 percent has been noted by Type I diabetic women.

If a diabetic woman wants to take estrogen and progesterone at the time of menopause, her insulin requirement will be affected. The insulin requirement will depend on how perfectly the hormone doses match her needs. High doses of estrogen and progesterone require larger doses of insulin than low doses of estrogen and progesterone.

June and Barbara: We've heard both pros and cons about hormonal replacement. Do you think it's a good idea?

Dr. Jovanovic: Recently, it has been reported that estrogen plays a major role in calcium metabolism. Menopausal women are predisposed to osteoporosis (brittle bones). Better research has also shown that when estrogens are combined with progesterones to mimic the normal menstrual cycle, there is no increase in cancer. With less of a cancer scare, more physicians prescribe estrogens and progesterones to menopausal women to treat depression, hot flashes, and skin and hair changes associated with menopause—and to assure that calcium metabolism is kept normal. Most physicians will rein-force a high-calcium diet of 1200 to 1500 mg of calcium per day along with the hormones to keep the bones sturdy.

June and Barbara: If a woman has a history of uterine or breast cancer, are estrogen and progesterone still considered okay?

Dr. Jovanovic: No. Many cancers of the breast, in partic-ular, are spread by estrogens. Although the tissue is usu-ally tested for the estrogen receptors, it is not okay for a woman with a history of previous cancer to take estro-gens because of the possibility that the cancer is sensitive to estrogens.

June and Barbara: It is very common for women—dia-betic or not—to find to their distress that after the meno-pause or a hysterectomy they gain a lot of weight. What's the reason for this?

Dr. Jovanovic: When a dog is spayed it becomes fat. Interesting, isn't it, since dogs don't have eating disor-ders! What this proves is that on one can of dog food a day, a dog that was lean and lovely before fixing can get fat and old after fixing. Therefore, to claim that a meno-pausal woman is getting fat because she "overeats" is a bit accusing. Actually, metabolism slows down by 25 per-cent after menopause, so unless the intake of food is decreased by 25 percent, the woman will gain weight.

June and Barbara: What a rotten deal! Can nothing be done about this? Can't we rev up our metabolism in some way? For example, several authors on weight loss —including Covert Bailey, of *Fit or Fat?* fame—maintain that you can change your metabolism through a program of regular vigorous exercise so that your body will burn more calories even when you're sitting still or sleeping.

Dr. Jovanovic: Not only can exercise metabolize glucose immediately but it also has a prolonged effect that may last up to twenty-four hours. So it is true that vigorous exercise for twenty minutes a day means more efficient fuel-burning for the rest of the day. Therefore, with exercise a woman can reverse that problem of burning 25 percent fewer calories.

June and Barbara: The psychological problems that occur after menopause and in later life can be even more devastating than the physiological ones. Could you offer diabetic women some help and guidance in coping with these?

Dr. Jovanovic: It's natural to grieve that you are growing older. Joints creak, a familiar flight of stairs seems to suddenly have more steps, the midline enlarges, the skin dries and wrinkles, and the hair turns gray and falls out. These physical changes certainly can be depressing for any woman, but a woman with diabetes may also perceive that she is somehow growing old *faster* than a nondiabetic friend the same age. Actually, high blood sugars do dry and scale the skin, change the vaginal secretions, and make the nails deteriorate. We used to be taught in medical school that diabetes makes people look ten years older than their chronological age. But better glucose control can slow down the aging process so that we diabetic women can suffer just like everyone else.

When a woman with diabetes goes through menopause, the emotional changes may lead to a deterioration in control. Deterioration in control increases aging, which leads to more depression. The best way for a woman to prevent this is to share the problem with a responsible diabetes health-care professional, who can take over her insulin adjustments until she is psychologically ready to take back her self-care.

Depression does *not* lead to the motivation to care about self-care. An understanding health-care professional will be able to unload the diabetes care from the woman, thus allowing her to have more energy to cope with her other problems. Perhaps even a few sessions with a psychologist to learn coping skills would be helpful.

Exercise can be the perfect prescription for this depression. Exercise reverses the midline bulge, increases energy levels, and produces endorphins. Endorphins are naturally occurring brain substances that make us feel happy. These substances are responsible for the "runner's high," a feeling of euphoria much like the feeling one gets from taking an upper, or pep pill. In addition, exercise burns sugar and can therefore be used to improve glucose control.

But exercise does not immediately feel good. In fact, in an unfit person, strenuous exercise is actually stressful and potentially harmful. Becoming fit requires a step-by-step program. One suggested program would be as follows:

Three times a week, an hour should be set aside for your exercise. This would be composed of ten minutes of warm-up and stretching, followed by twenty minutes of aerobics. This would be any exercise that keeps the pulse in the training range, such as bicycle riding, running, or jumping rope. To find your training pulse range, subtract your age in years from 220, then multiply the result by 70 percent. For example, a fifty-year-old woman would need to maintain a pulse rate of 119 for twenty minutes. For a twenty-year-old woman this means a pulse of 140 for twenty minutes. When a woman is not fit, it takes only a little effort to bring the pulse up to the training range. As the program increases fitness, the amount of exertion needed to get the pulse up to the training range increases. After six months, the heart should be fit.

The aerobic exercise should be followed by twenty minutes of gentle cool-down exercise.

The last ten minutes of the hour should be used for a shower.

Ideally, the program should be done in a gym with an exercise physiologist who can teach the exercises, take the pulse, and increase the exertion level gradually.

In addition, a woman with diabetes should measure her blood sugar before the exercise program to ensure that it is 100–180 mg/dl. Starting an exercise program with a blood sugar of much lower than 100 does not leave room to burn up sugar. Either the exercise should be rescheduled for the next day and the insulin dose decreased, or twenty grams of carbohydrate should be eaten.

Exercising when the blood sugar is high only makes the sugar go higher. The exercise physiologist should be trained in blood-sugar checking and treatment of an insulin reaction.

Once a woman is fit and knows what exercises to perform, then she may continue the program on her own to stay fit—and euphoric—for the rest of her life.

June and Barbara: Some of the happiest pieces of news on the exercise front came out of a study of 17,000 Harvard alumni, which revealed that you don't need to do exhausting things like running marathons to reap the life-saving benefits of exercise. Men who pursued such moderate activities as walking, climbing stairs, and participating in sports that used 2000 or more calories per week had death rates one-quarter to one-third lower than their more sedentary counterparts. The benefits of exercise peaked at 3500 calories per week; burning more calories than that proved slightly detrimental in some cases.

We're often asked, "What's the best exercise for a diabetic?" We think Dr. Howard F. Hunt, chairman of the Department of Physical Education at the University of California, San Diego, had a good answer for that one. He says, "The best exercise for a diabetic is the one he or she will do." How right he is! No matter how great someone else thinks an exercise is, if you find it boring, disgusting, or exhausting you're not going to do it. So you should shop around among sports activities until you find one that inspires you to action.

One activity that most people enjoy—and that does not take any special equipment, can be done anywhere, and doesn't cause physical damage—is walking. You almost can't walk too much. Of course, you must walk with a certain amount of vigor for the cardiovascular benefit. But rigorous walking is something you can work up to by starting slowly and gradually increasing your pace until the significant day that you make the fifteen-minute mile.

Dr. Lawrence Power recently sang the praises of walking in his syndicated newspaper column: "A group of overweight volunteers were placed on restricted diets of 1000 calories a day. Half also were put on a 30-minute-a-day walking program; the other half were not. . . . All subjects were measured at the start and finish for total body fat and muscle. The walking group had gained two pounds of muscle and lost 25 pounds of fat. The non-walking group had lost eight pounds of muscle and 12 pounds of fat."

Dr. Power also pointed out that the diet-only group gained back weight much more easily than the diet-and-exercise group, thanks to their smaller muscle mass. That's because muscle is a "metabolically busy" tissue and burns more calories than fat.

There's another exercise that's even easier to fit into your life than walking. It can literally be done anywhere, except maybe in a phone booth. It's called "jarming"—jogging for the arms. To really get your heart pumping, just swing your arms around as vigorously as if you were conducting the Boston Pops playing the 1812 Overture. It's a great way to sneak in a little exercise in the middle of your workday—and you're bound to work more efficiently with all that exercise-generated oxygen flooding your brain. Our theory is that the reason symphony conductors live to such ripe old ages is that they spend their careers jarming. We admit that our theory lacks scientific validity. As you know from diabetes research, the only studies taken seriously are done with rats. And it's hard to get rats to stand around swinging their arms all day.

Besides longevity, jarming promotes a youthful aura. *Cosmopolitan*'s Helen Gurley Brown says that the best indicator of a woman's aging is loose flesh in the upper arm. One way to make your jarming even more effective is to wear Aerobic Rings on your wrists or hold onto Heavy Hands: both are weights that build strength and burn calories. Using these in conjunction with walking gives you a total exercise treatment.

One woman wrote us asking for information on heart disease, saying, "Some troublesome symptoms I experienced for some time were mistakenly attributed by my doctor to bouts of low blood sugar. (When I began testing blood-sugar levels, I found this was *not* so!) Then, almost by serendipity, I found that the chest pains and irregular heart were due to a not-so-innocent mitral valve prolapse [MVP]. MVP is usually considered 'harmless,' whereas the version I have is a progressive form that greatly increases the work of the heart."

Is the mitral valve prolapse likely to have been caused by her diabetes?

Dr. Jovanovic: Mitral valve prolapse is a separately inherited disease. Thus, the woman who wrote this letter inherited both MVP and diabetes mellitus. Diabetes does cause premature atherosclerosis, however, when the sugar level is sustained above normal for years. In fact, the usual statement is that diabetes "equalizes" the prevalence of atherosclerotic causes of heart attack. In other words, a diabetic woman would have the same chances of having a heart attack at the same age as a nondiabetic man. A nondiabetic woman has only a 5 percent chance of having a heart attack before menopause, whereas a woman who has had diabetes for more than thirty years has a 50 percent chance of this.

June and Barbara: Those are rather discouraging statistics, but we've always had the theory that diabetes can, in some ways, be beneficial to your health. For example, a fifty-year-old diabetic woman who understands healthy living and takes good care of herself could conceivably be in better shape than a twenty-year-old nondiabetic who's let herself go to pot through ignorance and sloth. Have you seen evidence of this in your practice?

Dr. Jovanovic: Unfortunately, I have seen unfit, fat women who can barely climb a flight of steps without becoming short of breath. But fortunately, I have seen many diabetic women over the age of fifty who are fit and a picture of health. I have personally met two elderly women who received the Joslin Medal for fifty years of diabetes with no evidence of any complications. Any of our readers who have had diabetes for fifty years and who are in good health should apply for the medal. (Write to the Joslin Diabetes Foundation, 50 Joslin Road, Boston, MA 02215.)

CHAPTER
3

BOTH SIDES NOW

Oh wad some power the giftie gie us
To see oursels as others see us!
                    —Robert Burns

Now that we've looked at the picture of diabetes from your point of view, we're going to "gie you the giftie" of seeing it from the perspective of those close to a diabetic woman. We hope that their words will help you to help your family and friends come to terms with situations that may hurt and disturb them as much as—or more than—they hurt and disturb you. We suggest that after reading these sections, you pass them on to the appropriate people in your life.

Dr. Peterson (Dr. Jovanovic's husband), who tells the following story, is an eminent endocrinologist and coauthor of *The Diabetes Self-Care Method*.

LOVE, LIFE, AND THE PURSUIT OF HAPPINESS WITH A DIABETIC WOMAN

Charles M. Peterson, M.D.

What happens when the woman you love has diabetes? Well, if it occurs during your relationship, you tend to deny it until that doesn't work, then you get angry and ask, "Why us?" and finally you begin to acquire better coping skills—but only after a time of real depression.

How can two people who have been to medical school and who specialize in diabetes deny that one of them has the disease? Easily. It hurts too much to accept it all at once, no matter how "smart" you may be. The hurt does not go away very soon, either.

One of the best things that families in which someone has developed diabetes can do is talk with someone about the experience and about diabetes itself. The format is almost not as important as the process, since talking helps overcome denial and helps move the family through the stages of grief into the real world of coping. Unfortunately, the male of the species is less apt to talk with others about the real hurts of life and more likely to keep them inside. In addition, his soul mate is the one with diabetes—and he feels it would be better if it were he. Certainly, it is easier to cope with your own infirmities —physical and spiritual—than with those of the one you love.

Which brings us to the next problem: a man likes action; he likes to fix things and make them right—preferably *now*. Yet there is no way for a man to fix his partner's diabetes. He has to let her grow, make mistakes, and suffer with her own diabetes without interfering with the process and yet be there to discuss, support, and learn with her. It is difficult to let go of children so they can grow, but it is even more difficult to let go of a spouse who has a chronic illness. Diabetes is a time of taking hold and setting free, just like marriage itself.

Yet you *can* take away some of your own anxiety so that you can help your partner in more and deeper ways. Anxiety comes from the unknown, so learn to cope with diabetes. (It will take a lifetime to learn to cope with your partner anyway, so start with the diabetes—it's easier!) Learn about measuring blood sugar. Practice on yourself. Learn about injections by giving yourself injections of sterile saline [salt solution]. Learn how to inject glucagon to bring her out of a hypoglycemic episode, and have a plan to ensure that you will always have glucagon available where both of you can find it. Once in Italy I did the world's fastest and messiest unpacking job at 3 A.M., because we were too lazy to locate the glucagon before going to bed after the flight from the United States. It took us about two hours to get the room in shape the next morning so we wouldn't be embarrassed when the maid saw it.

Learn about food and the carbohydrate count of various foods so that you can help her count carbos, and you will both begin to have a healthier eating pattern. Learn about exercise (strength training, cardiovascular conditioning, and flexibility) and start a program for both of you.

Families get stronger from coping with challenges. Cope with the challenge of diabetes as a family. If you seem to be stuck, get a consultation from a professional. Above all, keep learning, growing, and challenging each other so that you as a family are taking charge of diabetes and winning over it—with love.

June and Barbara: We've seen the truth of all of Dr. Peterson's words in action. Amy's husband, Michael, became such an expert in diabetes during her pregnancy that now whenever he meets someone in his business who has diabetes in the family, he gives them an instant education. He takes a great deal of pride in being able to help others in this way. And we've often seen how the health and vitality of a family improves when the whole family adopts the lifestyle of its diabetic member.

Unfortunately, not all husbands are like Dr. Peterson and Michael, as this letter from Karen Kremsreiter in Baraboo, Wisconsin, points out.

My husband was very supportive. He read every piece of literature I brought home and helped me figure out dietary calculations. He learned how to give me shots in places I thought I couldn't reach. (I've since learned to inject myself anywhere.) He learned how to use glucagon and often recognized signs of an insulin reaction long before I did. Looking back (I'm forty years old now), I feel that my husband's support and involvement were critical in my ability to become confident and adept in diabetes management.

Although he is no longer so intensely involved with my routine, he is still willing to listen and learn. That means that there is one person (aside from my doctor) with whom I can have an intelligent conversation about diabetes and who understands the fine points of diabetes management.

The reason I mention my husband's support is that I see this kind of support lacking among the majority of diabetic women I meet. When a diabetes support group started in my town about ten years ago, I was eager to join. My husband went to meetings with me, and we both learned a lot. However, we were surprised to find so few men at these meetings. I assumed that there weren't many diabetic men in my town (wrong!) or that some of the elderly women were widowed (wrong again!).

Eventually, I became chairman of the diabetes group, which gave me the chance to get to know the members well. Over the years, the patterns have remained pretty much the same. Husbands generally do not attend meetings with their diabetic wives. However, wives usually do attend with their diabetic husbands, or wives attend FOR their husbands or diabetic children. The woman, it seems, is still considered the primary caretaker of the health of all family members.

The sad part of this pattern is that women who have supportive husbands (or sisters or friends) do much better, healthwise. The diabetic women who attend meetings alone seem to have many more complaints about stress. They worry that their diabetes is "inconveniencing" their husbands and families. They require more trips to the doctor and need to ask for rides to meetings they wish to attend. Many of these women seem to develop complications of diabetes sooner.

Women need to be convinced that they never have to apologize to anyone for having diabetes. Moreover, they should insist that another family member learn some fine points of diabetes care. Type II diabetes, especially, is often glossed over as a mild, harmless disorder by other family members. It's time people realized that Type II diabetes can be as fatal as Type I diabetes when the home treatment is sloppy and inadequate. Diabetes care requires a lot of education and some special techniques, which all family members should be involved in. And a woman should not feel guilty for placing her health above other family problems.

Any suggestions you can make for involving husbands and family members in the diabetes management program would be helpful. Perhaps it is the family doctor who needs to be more aggressive in involving the entire family.

Dr. Jovanovic: Mrs. Kremsreiter is correct about the fact that women who have support at home do better. Studies have clearly shown that when a husband and wife are in conflict about the diabetes, her hemoglobin A_1C is the highest.

I also agree with her about the family doctor's responsibility for involving the family. He or she could use glucagon-injection education as a gimmick to force the husband to come into the office, and once he is there a bit of family therapy could be started. This should be followed up with an appointment with a real family therapist who is trained in diabetes.

June and Barbara: Perhaps you could also provide us with a few guidelines on setting up a support group, so that women out there alone could actually initiate a network if none existed in the community.

Dr. Jovanovic: That's very possible. Anyone can start a support group. When people with the same problems meet together spontaneously, things get better. Even without a professional counselor to guide discussions, the group process is helpful, because just living with diabetes means that coping skills have been developed. Thus an experienced person with diabetes can do wonders for a new diabetic.

The group can benefit, too, from a professionally trained person with skills in coping, but not having such an expert should in no way deter you from starting a support group.

June and Barbara: Both you and Dr. Peterson point out the necessity of getting psychological help from a professional if you seem to be stuck. This is tremendously valid. We should all get rid of that old Sam Goldwyn idea that anybody who goes to a psychiatrist ought to have his head examined. No one should ever hesitate to seek psychological counseling when it's called for. Nancy Slonim Aronie, the mother of a diabetic child, gave a vivid example of how effective such counseling can be by relating the following personal experience on National Public Radio's program "All Things Considered."

THE NIGHT MOM LOST IT AT FRIENDLY'S

Nancy Slonim Aronie

I used to think I would never go to a psychologist. Psychologists were for the rich, the spoiled, and the bored, and, of course, the crazy. I prided myself on being none of these. Then when my nine-month-old son was diagnosed as diabetic, my life changed. His diabetes didn't make me rich, spoiled, or bored, but it almost made me crazy. I had to give him two shots of insulin a day in his tiny little arms. I had to collect his urine in little plastic bags and test it for sugar three times a day. I worried when he was napping that he would never wake up, and I worried in the middle of the night whether he had eaten enough before he went to sleep.

When he got a little older, other parents worried. He soon learned he held this terrible power. Grown-ups were afraid of him. They would ask him what he wanted, and if he needed to rest, and if he were thirsty, and what should they make special for him when he was coming over to play with their children. He didn't like this power, and they didn't like having a kid visiting who might die on them any minute. His invitations were limited. As parents we tried very hard not to indulge him . . . to treat him like a "normal" person. But every so often we blew it.

One night after a concert we took our two kids out to Friendly's and he asked for ice cream. I said no. My husband said, "Oh, let him have ice cream."

"LET HIM?!" I screamed, "Oh, I get it. *I'm* in charge of the pancreas. *I* can make it work. *I'm* the bad guy here, and you're the good guy. Poor Dan. He never gets a treat, and it's my fault."

At this point in my life I had many psychologist friends who had erased the myth that therapy was lying on a couch once a week for fourteen years while a Freudian-looking shrink with pencil poised in hand nodded and told you all your problems stemmed from the fact that you were really in love with your father, hated your mother, and wished you were your brother. So I called a few of my friends and said, "this diabetes thing has gotten out of hand. Dan is angry all the time, and I am guilty all the time, and we need help. Whom should we go see?"

I got a name, and within a week the four of us were sitting in an office in four big leather chairs in a circle.

The doctor asked my eleven-year-old son, "Why are you here?"

"I think it's because of the night my mom lost it at Friendly's," he said.

The doctor turned to my nine-year-old, the one with diabetes, and said, "Why do *you* think you're here?"

My nine-year-old smiled and said, "Yup, that's it. It was the night my mom lost it at Friendly's."

And then he turned to my husband, who had fought tooth and nail not to go to this appointment. My husband nodded in agreement. "Yeah. We're here because Nance made us come."

Then the doctor turned to me. I reached for the box of Kleenex on his desk and burst into tears. I said, "We're here because this child thinks the world is going to change its rules for him because he has diabetes. *He* gets four strikes in baseball, not three. And this child, who doesn't have diabetes, is wounded because all of the focus has been on the other one. And this man, my husband, doesn't want a child with diabetes because it hurts too much. So I'm the only one who has a son with diabetes, and they all think I control the pancreas, and, please, could you shape us up in short order?"

The doctor smiled and asked some key questions. We told a story of how one night before a fancy party I had prepared my son with a lecture on how there would be all these tempting foods, telling him that he should have a small amount of everything so that he wouldn't feel deprived.

The first person to grab a plate was my son, and when I saw the huge mound of sweet-potato pudding he had taken, I said, "Dan, I thought we had talked about having small portions of everything."

"This *IS* small!" he screamed, then smashed the plate down and ran out of the room crying.

The doctor gave a great analogy. He said to Dan, "If you were describing a quarter to a kid who was poor and you were describing the same quarter to a kid who was rich, how would the rich kid's understanding of the size of the quarter be different from the poor kid's?"

Dan said, "Well, the rich kid would see the quarter smaller because a quarter isn't much money to him, but to a poor kid a quarter is a lot so it would be bigger."

"Exactly," said the doctor. "Well, to your mom, who worries about your health because she loves you, the amount of sweet-potato pudding was a lot, but to you, who never has enough, the pudding portion was small."

I saw my son understand. I saw the switch go on. I saw him see that all I was doing was loving him and worrying about him, not trying to make his life miserable.

The next session we talked about his anger. The doctor said, "Your mom didn't give you diabetes. She's sorry you have diabetes. It's not fair, but life isn't fair. Your mom is not in charge of your pancreas. Neither is your father or your brother. Being angry is okay, but choose where the anger goes. Your mother is hurting, and she loves you. Being angry at her is not going to make the diabetes go away."

Another click. Another light. A few more sessions and the doctor told us to go home and to call if we had a crisis or just wanted to come in and talk.

Now there is harmony in my house except for the usual teenage growing-up stuff, and I realize what a luxury it is to be able to go and talk to a pro and get perspective so simply, so easily, so quickly. It takes work. It takes commitment (and a willingness to change and to hear some truths), but you don't have to be rich, spoiled, bored, or crazy—and you can even go talk to someone *before* you lose it at Friendly's.

This story shows the problems a mother can have in coping with her child's diabetes, but probably the most difficult moment for the mother comes when the child— particularly a very young child—is diagnosed as diabetic. What do you say and do to help a mother at this time?

Dr. Jovanovic: I have thought about this question for a long while, because my experience with mothers of diabetic children is limited. As you know, I am an internist, which means that I take care of adults. My youngest patients are twelve years old, but I treat them as adults, and my interaction with their parents is minimal.

Yes, I have given numerous lectures to parents of diabetic children, but this formal setting does not lend itself to answering intimate questions. Usually these parent groups are composed of experienced parents who just want to learn more about diabetes research. I really could not answer this question with the voice of experience until just recently, when I came face to face with it on a very personal level.

A childhood friend of mine with whom I had not communicated for years called me up. She is a very special person of whom I was always envious. She succeeded in becoming the prima ballerina of the New York City Ballet Company, whereas I was too short and too awkward to make it as a ballerina, so I became a doctor. Not only is she truly talented and exquisitely beautiful, but she is also blessed with a beautiful personality. This is all to tell you that there never was a more perfect woman created. Why, then, did diabetes strike her one-year-old daughter?

Two weeks before she telephoned me, her daughter had been taken to the hospital in diabetic coma. I heard her pain and grief. Her emotions were mixed with anger and disbelief. To make matters worse, no one at the hospital helped her to cope, grieve, and begin to accept. No one told her what diabetes is, what it meant for her daughter, and what the best management program is. My friend left the hospital with her daughter out of coma, but with no understanding of how to give insulin and how to prepare meals. I just listened and grieved with her. It is quite possible that the best diabetes educator tediously went over all the basics, but one thing is sure. The week the little one is on the critical list is no time to try to teach skills that take complete attention.

My response was not to take sides but instead to offer a sympathetic ear. No, God was not punishing her. Goodness knows that she, of all people, did not deserve punishment. Yet her sense of guilt was real, and my job was to tell her over and over that diabetes occurs spontaneously. If sin caused diabetes, it would be easier to cure.

My next job was to direct her to support systems. I referred her to a specialized center for children with diabetes that has a team whose members are expert on the problems children face. The dietitian is skilled in baby food, the psychologist knows how to handle baby problems, and the diabetes doctor knows baby metabolism. In addition, my friend could meet other mothers and share experiences. She could also take classes to learn more about diabetes. This would help her not to feel so inadequate.

My last job was to reassure her that I was overjoyed about renewing our friendship and that I was here for her. Too often, friends tend to shy away when there are problems, and it is at this time that support is most needed.

A week later my friend called me again. Her voice was full of hope. She had learned insulin action, and her fear of hypoglycemia was not constantly present. She had learned how to do blood tests to prevent hypoglycemia, and she had learned how to treat hypoglycemia. She then confessed that her fear of hypoglycemia was greater than her fear of the diagnosis of diabetes. The psychologist solved this problem easily. The dietitian spoke in ways that made sense for feeding a year-old baby. The diabetes doctor developed better doses of insulin, which matched the eating and sleeping patterns of a small child. Life seemed better. But I explained to my friend that accepting the diagnosis of diabetes takes at least a year and that it certainly is not an indulgence to grieve.

June and Barbara: You mentioned the anger of your friend over her child's diabetes. We see this all the time. In fact, we find that possibly the angriest people on the face of the earth are the mothers of diabetic children. In his book *Feeling Good,* Dr. David Burns writes that one of the greatest sources of anger is the feeling that a situation is unfair. And what could be more unfair than having your innocent child, who has never done anything to anyone, be diagnosed as diabetic? Psychoanalyst Willard Gaylen believes that one cause of anger is the feeling of not having control over a situation. Both are probably right.

A big problem with anger, however, is that diabetics and parents of diabetics often don't like to admit, even to themselves, that the source of their anger is diabetes. So they displace their anger, directing it toward something or someone else. You may have experienced this yourself. Perhaps you have suddenly become furious over the time you've had to spend in the waiting room, over the doctor's bill, about the meter that reads a high number, or even with the well-meaning and compassionate health professional who is trying to help you make changes that you don't want to make. This last is a prime cause of burnout and compassion fatigue among diabetes health professionals. Even though they try to understand the reasons behind your anger, it really breaks their hearts and spirits when you suddenly and without provocation bite their helping hands.

The worst thing about displacing your anger—even worse than the psychic damage you do to a hapless "displacee"—is that if you never admit the true source of your anger, you'll never get rid of it. It will keep festering and then erupting. As Gaylen puts it, "Expressing anger is a form of public littering . . . how futile and how dangerous it is." He also shoots down the idea that it's therapeutic to let off steam by blowing up. It is far better to permanently resolve the situation that is the source of your anger. Again, some kind of therapy may be needed to do this.

The one good thing we can say about anger is that it's a step up from depression, which some experts regard as inner-directed anger and an even harder problem to deal with.

Another prime source of anger and also of resentment (which we have heard defined as a demand that someone feel guilty) is the situation in which one member of the family, such as a child, has diabetes, and the others do not. Should everyone be made to eat only what the diabetic child can? Should the child's brothers and sisters just ignore the diabetes? How much special attention should the diabetic child get?

Dr. Jovanovic: The brothers and sisters of a diabetic child should not be deprived of the delights of cakes, candies, sodas, chocolates, and ice cream. All too often, if siblings are denied things, they become angry and resentful of the diabetic child. Perhaps it is better to teach the diabetic child about the real world, which is full of forbidden foods, but to do so gently. For example, I usually suggest that whenever the family is on an outing and the other kids get an ice cream cone, the child with diabetes could have an alternative snack (yogurt, hot dog, popcorn) and should also get an extra treat—say, a toy—that the others do *not* get.

All of the brothers and sisters should be taught to be comfortable with diabetes, needles, and blood tests. The diabetes should not be hidden from the rest of the family; rather, the process of diabetes care should be shared. I like to suggest that the premeal blood-glucose strip be read visually by all the other children, with the one who reads it closest to the meter reading getting something special.

Many times the other brothers and sisters feel left out and are in fact jealous of the doted-on diabetic child. Here, the mother needs to be sensitive to these feelings, and she should try to spend as much special time with each of the other children as she does with the diabetic child.

The hardest job for mom is not to be overly protective. Except for insulin injections, a diabetic child is no different physically or mentally from other children, and he or she should therefore not be treated as a crippled person. Too often the child will succumb to a lazy dependence, and the growing-up process becomes more difficult than it ought to be. The mother needs to be brave, allowing the child independence and the right to make mistakes. Gentle guidance can be used to right the wrong and reinforce the right. I guess we are asking mom to be a saint—but after all, diabetes only happens to the best people!

June and Barbara: It's important for parents of diabetic children to go out in order to get out from under the strain of caring for a diabetic child. However, they often worry all evening that the baby-sitter won't know what to do if there's a crisis. Do you have any suggestions for them?

Dr. Jovanovic: I've heard of parents of diabetic children doing baby-sitting trade-offs with parents of other diabetic children. I think this is a super idea. Then they can go out with confidence, knowing that their child is in the hands of someone who understands diabetes as only the parent of a diabetic child can. Diabetic moms make great baby-sitters, too!

June and Barbara: Some mothers who have diabetes wonder what they should tell their children about diabetes. Could you share with us your personal experience with your own children?

Dr. Jovanovic: My children need to accept me for what I am—a woman with diabetes. My diabetes doesn't make me unfair, dishonest, selfish, or uncaring. Yes, it does mean that I am less than perfect, and my children either love me anyway or they don't. The simplest thing to tell you is that if I am embarrassed about my diabetes, then so are my children. If I am open about my diabetes and make it a natural part of life, then I should not be surprised that my kids tell strangers that their mommy has diabetes. Not only are they not embarrassed, but they may also even be proud because mom is somehow special, or they may feel that they are special because they have so much medical background at a young age.

Five years ago I was invited to give a talk to first-year medical students to help in trying to create a new generation of doctors who would be more open to diabetes self-care. These med students were fresh out of college and probably didn't even know what insulin was. My five- and six-year-old children were not yet in school and my baby-sitter was sick, so I took my children to the lecture and sat them in the back with strict orders to be quiet.

I started the lecture and fell into my usual jargon of medicalese. I noted that the class was unruly, but I kept right up with my rushed pace in order to pack in as much information as possible, using the longest words. I spotted my six-year-old son walking down the aisle and climbing onto the stage. I continued to talk, but boy, was I mad! My son marched up to the podium and said, "Mommy, no one understands you. The people around me are muttering that they don't know what diabetes is."

I turned to my son and began my lecture over again. This time I tried to explain myself so *he* would understand. Every time I accidentally used a big word, he would stop me and ask for an explanation. At the end of the talk, he received a standing ovation. Now he joins me every year and we reenact this routine, to the joy of the students.

How did he know so much? How did he know where I should put the emphasis and what is important to teach? He knew because he grew up with a mom who has diabetes and who is open to him about needles and blood tests and about what to expect when I am hypoglycemic. When I have low blood sugar, I get irritated for no reason. He now knows me well enough not to ask, "Are you low?" because he knows that I will say, "I am NOT LOW." Instead, he asks me to do simple arithmetic. I happen to be quick at mental gymnastics, and if I have trouble with 99 minus 13, then even I will admit that I must be low. If I need him to help me eat or get food, he knows exactly what to do.

Teaching the children about diabetes is an everyday process and makes mothering special.

Novelist and philosopher Aldous Huxley spent his entire life in pursuit of knowledge. In his later years someone asked him, considering all his scholarship and deep thought, what philosophical conclusion he had reached. He paused. "I think," he said slowly, "it's just that we should all be a little kinder to one another."

The caring kindness given to a diabetic woman by those closest to her enriches their lives as much as it enriches hers.

And so it comes to pass that people who share an orbit with a woman who is special because of her diabetes become special themselves. In a sense they become almost Godlike because, to end as we began, on a Robert Burns note, "The heart benevolent and kind, The most resembles God."

CHAPTER
4

DIABETIC DIET
À LA CARTE

In using this title, we're not just continuing with the French motif. We're also pointing out a major change in the diabetic's eating plan. Back in the bad old days, every diabetic was handed a one-sheet exchange list of permitted foods—the diabetic menu. No substitutions. No variations. No accounting for individual tastes or ethnic preferences. The list was both boring and limited, and it was little wonder that most diabetics decided to forget the whole thing and just go back to eating what they wanted.

Mercifully, the boring, rigid menu for diabetics is gone forever. Even the American Diabetes Association /American Dietetic Association's *Exchange Lists for Meal Planning* were dramatically revised in 1986 to reflect the new theories on the diabetes diet (higher carbohydrate, higher fiber, lower sodium, and so on). But above and beyond that you'll find it is now possible for you to dine à la carte, choosing what pleases you, adjusting the diabetic diet to yourself rather than adjusting yourself to the diabetic diet. You do have to know what you're doing, though, and the best way to do this is to have an appointment or two with a dietitian who can help you create an eating plan that is compatible both with your taste and with the requirements of your diabetes. You'll be amazed at how close these two can be.

Armed with this knowledge, you can play infinite variations on your particular diabetic eating-plan theme. Appendix A lists an array of cookbooks that promise you can dine like a gourmet, feast like a queen, and enjoy all manner of international cuisines. These books live up to their promises.

Even restaurants are featuring the healthier, lighter nouvelle, California, and Southwestern cuisines. Heavy sauces oozing butter and cream are out. It almost seems as though the whole world has suddenly discovered the diabetic diet, and those of us who have been following it for years find that we've been in the avant-garde. We former dietary outcasts now find ourselves insiders. It's just as we keep saying: If you had to go and get diabetes, you couldn't have picked a better time to do it!

In case you don't have access to a dietitian to get you started down the right gastronomic paths, we'll ask Dr. Jovanovic to give you advice on weight loss or weight gain, as well as a brief rundown of the basics of the best kinds of eating plans for the different types of diabetes. Then we'll follow up with some tips of our own, along with tips from our male diabetic diabetes dietitian, Ron Brown.

June and Barbara: Women in our society are, unfortunately, overly concerned with their weight for appearance' sake. Along with the natural human tendency to want to look good in society's terms, diabetic women also have the need to keep their weight at a healthy level. Often, we see Type I women who need to put on a few pounds and Type II women who need to take off a few

—or many—pounds. Why is there this difference? Let's take the Type Is first.

Dr. Jovanovic: A Type I diabetic running high blood sugars usually has an intense feeling of hunger, known medically as polyphasia. The added calories she tends to eat at this time are usually lost into the urine. Therefore, classically out-of-control diabetes in an insulin-dependent woman is usually associated with cachexia (being markedly underweight).

Once the diabetes is brought under control, the calories no longer spill over into the urine. Instead, the body, with the help of insulin, stores the extra calories in the form of fat. Unfortunately, after a time of overeating, the natural habit will be to continue to overeat even if calories are no longer being lost into the urine. For that reason, you have to make a major effort to decrease caloric intake along with following any program of tightening blood-sugar control.

In addition, many women swell up when they come into better control. Diabetes out of control is associated with thirst from massive urination. Even though the massive urination stops when the diabetes is in better control, the habit to overdrink remains. Thus, an effort to decrease fluid intake to one quart a day helps prevent this swelling.

June and Barbara: That's an important point about fluid intake. One Type I diabetic woman who got herself in good control was disturbed by abdominal bloating. What confused her—and us—was that she was not at all overweight, yet she had developed a distended stomach. Apparently, she had cut back on her calories to keep her weight normal, but she didn't realize that she was still drinking as many fluids as ever.

We hate to mention the following because we don't want to give anyone any bad ideas, but if a Type I diabetic woman wanted to lose weight she could just get out of control again by decreasing her insulin, and no matter what she ate she wouldn't gain weight.

Dr. Jovanovic: Yes, the extra calories would automatically come out into the urine. This is what we call "diabetic anorexia," and it would be as damaging to the diabetic woman as the other anorexia—in fact, even more so. Not only would she have the poor health risks of being too thin, this terrible blood-sugar control would put her at risk for the horrifying complications of diabetes and, if carried to an extreme, for ketoacidosis and death.

When a woman is in good control, she realizes that it takes willpower to diet and exercise in order to stay fit. She also realizes that it's worth the effort, since her reward will be to look and feel wonderful now and to avoid complications later on in life.

June and Barbara: How about the Type II women and their ongoing struggle to get weight off? We have even heard that it might be said that in many Type II diabetic women the disease is obesity and that *this* is what needs to be treated. Their diabetes is considered to be a symptom of the disease of obesity. Is there a way to help these women lose weight? Would even the bad idea of staying out of control enable them to drop pounds?

Dr. Jovanovic: Not at all. A Type II woman stays fat when her diabetes is out of control. The reason for this is that her pancreas makes too much insulin, trying desperately to bring down the high blood sugar that builds up because of overeating. The large quantities of circulating insulin pack the calories away into fat cells. Giving insulin to these women packs away even more calories into fat, but the reason these women eat so much is that the high blood sugar causes increased hunger. If the added insulin can bring down the blood sugar, the hunger drive may let up some, but giving even more insulin to a person who already has too much of her own insulin doesn't make sense.

The treatment of choice, then, for a Type II woman is to decrease the food ingestion, which will in turn decrease the buildup of sugar in the bloodstream. But this isn't an easy treatment to carry out.

Most Type II diabetic women became obese from an eating disorder to begin with, and the obesity is what has brought out the diabetes—so in a sense the theory you mention about obesity's being the primary disease has some validity.

Since an eating disorder *is* involved, merely prescribing a diet is useless. A physician must provide, first, good educational support; second, a dietitian to translate the physician's prescription into meal planning; and third, psychological support—not only with trained psychologists specializing in eating disorders but also with group support such as Weight Watchers, Overeaters Anonymous, and so on, in which the patients help one another to sustain willpower. Physicians are not true to their patients if they think that all they need to do is write out a diet prescription and say, "See me in a month."

Thus, every woman with an eating disorder needs help, whether or not she has diabetes and, if so, whether the diabetes is Type I or Type II. The best help is obtained by seeing a clinical psychologist trained in eating disorders and by attending group help sessions with peer input.

June and Barbara: Weight loss is such a problem for many diabetic women that it would help a great deal if you could give a specific weight-loss program for Type Is and Type IIs. We assume these programs would be different. Let's start with the Type Is.

Dr. Jovanovic: For a Type I diabetic woman, the best way to go on a diet is to first become stabilized with the right amount of insulin to match the right amount of food for maintaining a steady body weight. Then, if the food intake is reduced by 25 percent, the insulin taken to cover the food can also be reduced by 25 percent. Let's say that the breakfast meal took eight units of regular, lunch took four units of regular, and dinner took eight units of regular. If each meal were reduced by 25 percent, then breakfast would require six units of regular, lunch three units of regular, and dinner six units of regular.

As far as diets are concerned, you have to be careful to *never* follow one of the popularized fad diets. These unbalanced "miracle weight-loss plans" that push one food—such as grapefruit—or one type of food (high protein, high fiber) to the exclusion of all others are bad enough for nondiabetics, but for diabetic people they are a disaster. The truth is that the only diets that produce a true weight reduction are those that cause you to lose the weight gradually by cutting the caloric intake below the caloric expenditure. (See Appendix A for recommended weight-loss books.)

To judge the amount of insulin needed, you must examine the particular diet, especially the amount of carbohydrate it contains. One unit of regular insulin covers about ten grams of carbohydrate. If food consists mostly of protein and fat, less insulin is needed. Fat does not need extra insulin to be metabolized. Protein is about 50 percent converted to glucose in about two or three hours. Therefore, protein usually is covered by the undercurrent basal insulin or the NPH or ultralente. Carbohydrate is covered by the mealtime regular.

I'll try to give a formula for figuring this: say, for example, that a woman weighing 60 kilograms (approximately 132 pounds) needs 0.6 units per kilogram to maintain normal blood sugar, with half of this insulin needed as the basal requirement and half needed for meals. Then, if the twenty-four-hour insulin requirement is represented by I: $I =$ Basal $+$ Mealtime Regular (or Basal $= \frac{1}{2}$ of I and Meals $= \frac{1}{2}$ of I).

If the meals equal 1800 calories (30 kcal $\times$ 60 kg) and 40 percent of this is carbohydrate, and if each gram of carbohydrate is 4 calories, then:

$$\frac{\text{GRAMS OF CARBOHYDRATE}}{24 \text{ HOURS}} = \frac{1800 \times 40\%}{4 \text{ CAL/GM CARBOHYDRATE}}$$

$$\text{OR}$$

$$= 180 \text{ GM CARBOHYDRATE PER } 24\text{-HOUR PERIOD}$$

IF THE MEALTIME REGULAR IS HALF OF I, THEN:

$$\frac{60 \text{ KG} \times 0.6}{2} = \frac{18 \text{ UNITS OF REGULAR COVER}}{180 \text{ GRAMS OF CARBOHYDRATE}}$$

If the meals are divided equally, then each meal has sixty carbohydrates and requires six units of insulin. Now you see why one unit of regular covers ten grams of carbohydrate.

On a diet *before* weight loss, the basal is still half of I per eighteen units until weight is lost, but the meal regular is decreased to intake. So if a person wants only twenty grams of carbohydrate for breakfast, she takes two units; for lunch, if she wants thirty grams of carbohydrate, she takes three units, and so on. Of course, a woman may find that for her one unit does not cover a full ten grams of carbohydrate, so she may need one unit for eight grams of carbohydrate. On the other hand, if she is sensitive to regular, she may take one unit of regular to cover twelve to fifteen grams of carbohydrate. With this match, food can be increased or decreased without hyperglycemia or hypoglycemia.

June and Barbara: Is it as complicated for a Type II diabetic?

Dr. Jovanovic: It's not as complicated, but it may be more difficult, because an overweight Type II may have "hungry fat cells" pleading for food all the time. The best plan is for these persons to have a constant support system. A program like Weight Watchers is most successful in giving support. Busy physicians are the worst support system, but they *are* needed to reduce the oral agents as needed while food intake and weight are decreased.

June and Barbara: We've heard a lot lately about fat cells being responsible for overweight, and the current medical tendency is to blame mothers for overfeeding babies and causing more fat cells to develop. Has this been proven, or is it just another case of the mother getting a bum rap?

Dr. Jovanovic: It hasn't yet been proven in humans, but they have discovered in laboratories that overfed baby rats develop more fat cells than their normally fed counterparts. Based on those studies, some researchers feel it would apply to people as well.

Other studies have found that overweight babies have larger-than-normal fat cells and also that very overweight adults have more than the normal number of fat cells. However, no one has yet discovered when this increase in fat cells occurs. They do know, however, that once a fat cell is formed, it's with you for life. It shrinks when you lose weight, but it's still there, fairly screaming with hunger. This helps to explain why people put back on as much weight as they have just lost or more. Their shrunken fat cells keep demanding food.

June and Barbara: We have a friend, a home-economics professor, who maintains that she'd be a perfect candidate for survival of enforced starvation because her body stores fat so efficiently and burns it off so inefficiently. Is this a common problem among overweight people?

Dr. Jovanovic: Yes, everyone's body has protective mechanisms that help protect it from starvation by changing the metabolism so that as much energy as possible is conserved. As soon as you cut back on food, the body adjusts itself to burning less.

June and Barbara: What's the answer, then, for overweight Type II women who have large fat cells and/or a "starvation-survival" metabolism?

Dr. Jovanovic: I'm afraid the answer is a dull one, and one you've heard a hundred times: a reduction in calories and an increase in exercise. Those weird crash diets may be easier to stick to because you figure you can stand anything for a brief period, but, almost invariably, as soon as the diet is over and the weight is lost you return to your old eating habits and put all the weight back on, usually with a few pounds' dividend. Not only that, but crash diets are usually unbalanced and unhealthy and therefore especially risky for a diabetic woman.

June and Barbara: A lot of women hesitate to quit smoking because it's almost axiomatic that you put on weight when you do. Why is this, and is there any way to keep it from happening?

Dr. Jovanovic: Smoking satisfies the oral needs. When a person stops smoking, she is withdrawing from a drug. The process is marked by irritability and nervousness, and some may be driven to nervous eating. The habits surrounding the lip and mouth movements are also satisfied by eating. They could just as well be satisfied by any chewing—even on a stick!

Yes, it takes willpower to stop smoking, but it takes even greater willpower not to turn to food as a comfort.

June and Barbara: Ron Brown, our dietitian at the Sugarfree Center, told us that when he is counseling diabetics about their diet he explains to them that Type Is need to be concerned mostly about the amount of carbohydrate they eat, and Type IIs about the amount of calories they eat. Do you agree with Ron on this, and could you elaborate?

Dr. Jovanovic: I think Ron is right, and that's certainly an easily understandable way of explaining the main dietary guidelines. Appropriate dietary recommendations, in my opinion, must always be based on the patient's type of diabetes. The ideal diet for one type of diabetes may worsen control in another type.

I would like to go into more detail about the amount of carbohydrate that is ideal for each type of diabetes. There has been a good deal of controversy recently in scientific circles about high-carbohydrate diets. The question is, are they beneficial for persons with diabetes or not? I think we can shed some light on this issue.

First, let's mention that the goal of diet is to help you maintain normal blood sugars, so the ideal diet for you is the one that facilitates keeping your blood sugars within the normal range. With this in mind, we can divide diabetic people into three distinctive categories.

1. Insulin-Dependent: Complete Pancreatic Insufficiency

If you are a Type I diabetic who produces no insulin of your own—we call this complete pancreatic insufficiency—then your problem is to calculate exactly how much insulin to inject to match the carbohydrate you eat. It is easier to match insulin with carbohydrate if you limit the total carbohydrate to 40 percent, most of which should be complex carbohydrate, high in fiber. Restricting carbohydrate to 40 percent will help you to avoid the roller-coaster effect: high blood glucose after you eat, and low blood glucose about three hours later, when your insulin peaks.

2. Insulin-Requiring: Partial Pancreatic Insufficiency

If you are insulin-requiring but your pancreas still secretes some insulin—partial pancreatic insufficiency—then restricting carbohydrate may not help your blood sugars. Since carbohydrate restriction decreases the amount of insulin your own pancreas secretes, it is advisable for you to eat as much as 70 percent carbohydrate, providing it is high in fiber. The higher percentage of carbohydrate will prime your own insulin-producing cells, and the fiber will slow down the conversion of carbohydrate into simple sugars. The end result will be blood sugars that are more consistently normal.

However, if you have difficulty matching your food to insulin when you eat 70 percent carbohydrate, then you are better off with 40 percent carbohydrate or maybe even a little less.

3. Non–Insulin-Requiring: Overweight

If you are an overweight Type II diabetic, then you need a restricted-calorie, restricted-carbohydrate diet. Again, complex carbohydrate high in fiber is advised. The lowered amount of carbohydrate will allow the insulin receptors of your cells to function normally instead of closing down, as they do when you overeat carbohydrate, stimulating your pancreas to overproduce insulin.

These dietary guidelines about the amount of carbohydrate to eat according to your type of diabetes are controversial. We have no proof yet as to whether their long-term effect will be beneficial. But in the interim, following these guidelines is the best choice.

As a final word I would add that diet prescription, in all cases, must be extremely individualized. You may prove to be an exception to any general dietary rule. Only your blood-sugar tests can tell you.

June and Barbara: Speaking of general dietary rules, in 1983 a new and also controversial one—the Glycemic Index—made all the newspapers. (Unfortunately, the stories garbled the findings somewhat, giving many diabetics the impression that they could—among other things—eat mounds of ice cream with nary a worry. Of course, *nobody*—diabetic or not—should eat mounds of ice cream!) While the research was based on too few people for definite conclusions to be drawn for everyone, it is an interesting and surprising study that has attracted a lot of attention in diabetes circles.

The Glycemic Index, which is basically a classification of how high and how fast the blood sugar is raised by individual carbohydrate foods, is the result of a study done by a team of researchers headed by Dr. David Jenkins of the University of Toronto. The index compares the way carbohydrate foods raise blood sugar with the way straight glucose raises it. Glucose, the form of sugar in the blood, is assigned an index number of 100.

Generally speaking, for a diabetic a low (slow-releasing) Glycemic Index food is preferred to a high (fast-releasing) Glycemic Index food. The chart below shows the Glycemic Index of some of the few foods that have been tested. (The small number of foods is one of the problems with the Glycemic Index.) However, Dr. Jenkins has warned that blood sugar is only one factor to consider. Calories and nutritional values count too. In other words, you cannot and should not eat by the Glycemic Index alone.

Some of the findings of the study are surprising. For example:

Some foods thought to cause a fast rise in blood sugar (apples, ice cream) cause only a gradual rise.

Some foods thought to cause a gradual rise (shredded wheat, carrots, potatoes) are really fast-releasing.

The form of the food can make a big difference. Instant potatoes are 80, while potato chips are only 51.

Fructose (in controlled diabetics) causes less of a blood-sugar increase than other simple sugars—only 20 percent as much as glucose.

Legumes (beans, peas) cause slow rises in blood sugar.

CARBOHYDRATE GLYCEMIC INDEX

Simple Sugars

Fructose—20	Honey—87
Sucrose—59	Glucose—100

Fruits

Apples—39	Bananas—62
Oranges—40	Raisins—64
Orange Juice—48	

Starchy Vegetables

Sweet Potatoes—48	Instant Potatoes—80
Yams—51	Carrots—92
Beets—64	Parsnips—97
White Potatoes—70	

Dairy Products

Skim Milk—32	Ice Cream—36
Whole Milk—34	Yogurt—36

Legumes

Soybeans—15	Garbanzos—36
Lentils—29	Lima Beans—36
Kidney Beans—29	Baked Beans—40
Black-Eyed Peas—33	Frozen Peas—51

Pasta, Corn, Rice, Bread

Whole-Wheat Pasta—42	White Bread—69
White Pasta—50	Whole-Wheat Bread—72
Sweet Corn—59	White Rice—72
Brown Rice—66	

Breakfast Cereals

Oatmeal—49	Shredded Wheat—67
All-Bran—51	Cornflakes—80
Swiss Muesli—66	

Miscellaneous

Peanuts—13	Sponge Cake—46
Sausages—28	Potato Chips—51
Fish Sticks—38	Mars Bars—68
Tomato Soup—38	

This chart indicates that the classic raiser of low blood sugar, orange juice, at forty-eight is not all that great. You'd be better off carrying around a pocketful of mashed potatoes or parsnips for diabetic hypoglycemic emergencies. Best of all, of course, is what we've always advocated: pure glucose tablets, such as Dextrosols. Topping off the Index at 100, they are the fastest, with the "mostest."

Incidentally, Phyllis Crapo, a dietitian who is a nationally recognized expert on the Glycemic Index, tells the story of how orange juice got its reputation as a treatment for insulin reactions. It seems that back when Banting and Best were conducting their initial experiments with insulin in Canada, their first patient was walking home after having had his insulin shot. He started to feel very strange, and he staggered to the door of the nearest house.

The woman answering the door looked at him, aghast. "My goodness, young man," she said, "you look *terrible!* Come inside and sit down. Let me give you a glass of orange juice."

He soon felt much better, and thus a tradition was born.

But back to the practicalities of the Glycemic Index. In your practice or your personal diet, have you found the Glycemic Index to be an accurate predictor of what will raise your blood sugar and of how fast it will do so?

Dr. Jovanovic: Although there are some general principles that apply to everyone, I've found that specific carbohydrates do different things to different people.

It's true that all persons with diabetes find that table sugar causes a higher, faster rise of the blood sugar than sorbitol, fructose, or lactose. However, all four of these sugars raise the blood sugar, and therefore you need extra insulin in order to consume them. How much more insulin is needed is specific to each person.

Yes, complex carbohydrates do absorb at different rates in different people. But whether rice, potato, bread, or pasta are the same or different is specific to each person. Therefore, each person needs to create a list of the relative strengths of each carbohydrate she eats. This would be a personal glycemic index.

Take me, for example. If my blood sugar is 100 mg/dl and I do not take regular insulin but instead let my blood sugar rise to show me the impact of different carbohydrates, then:

> 20 grams of bread raises my blood sugar to 300 at one hour
>
> 20 grams of rice raises my blood sugar to 270 at one hour
>
> 20 grams of cereal raises my blood sugar to 240 at one hour
>
> 20 grams of pasta raises my blood sugar to 240 at one hour
>
> 20 grams of bran raises my blood sugar to 200 at one hour

If each unit of regular insulin controls a rise of 25–30 mg/dl of blood sugar, and I do not want my blood sugar to go above 150 mg/dl, then I need:

> 6 units of regular for 20 grams of bread
>
> 5 units of regular for 20 grams of rice
>
> 4 units of regular for 20 grams of cereal
>
> 4 units of regular for 20 grams of pasta
>
> 2 units of regular for 20 grams of bran

The same experiment can be performed with simple sugars to find out how much insulin it takes to eat sweets!

June and Barbara: Phyllis Crapo agrees with you totally. She considers the Glycemic Index a general guideline, but she feels that it is best for each person to create her own personal glycemic index, as you have suggested.

June has done a number of tests along this line and finds that as far as her diabetes is concerned, the Glycemic Index is pretty accurate. In fact, it got to be a joke around the Sugarfree Center that if June had low blood sugar in the middle of the afternoon, we would always ask her if she had had pasta for lunch rather than a sandwich. Almost invariably, she had!

June has almost reached a point at which she runs in terror from cooked carrots and mashed potatoes, and she's found a true friend in sweet potatoes—something that in pre–Glycemic Index days she never ate, believing that because of their sweet taste they were forbidden.

The Glycemic Index has allowed other diabetics to add, with discretion, foods they formerly thought were denied them. Phyllis tells of a mother who came to her with tears of gratitude in her eyes because the Glycemic Index had revealed that ice cream was only 36 on the scale. The reason she was so delighted was because her little boy had been feeling tremendously deprived. A nightly dish of ice cream had been a family ritual that had to be dropped because of his diabetes. The Glycemic Index news had encouraged them to cautiously reintroduce ice cream into his life as his bedtime snack. Subsequent blood-sugar tests revealed that it didn't shoot up his blood sugar. She told Phyllis, "You can't imagine the difference a little dish of ice cream made in his life—and ours!" As a mother herself, Phyllis *could* imagine it.

We do find that sweets like ice cream are the hardest items in the diet for people to give up. Of course, if we were saints, we would eschew sweets of all kinds. Always. Under every circumstance. No exceptions. But, alas, we aren't saints.

As Dr. Lendon Smith writes in his foreword to the book *Sweet and Natural* (by Janet Warrington, Crossing Press, 1982), "Nature gave us taste buds to detect sweetness, and that sensory nerve goes right to the pleasure center of the brain."

One theory of our attraction to sweets is that back when our ancestors were, as you prefer, either swinging from trees or dwelling in the Garden of Eden, we needed to have vitamin C in our diets, so we were programmed to like the sweet taste of fruit.

But, for whatever reason, the fact remains that a sweet taste is something most of us like. We need to try to restrict it as much as possible and give our taste for sweets a chance to diminish, but on special occasions and for special treats it's a comfort to be able to have something special. Knowing that you can have an *occasional* sweet treat may keep you from going berserk and wolfing down a whole box of the bad stuff.

One thing that must be remembered about almost all diabetically possible sweet treats is that *they must be counted in your diet.* Beware of "sugar-free" candies and pastries and of bland assurances that you can eat as many of these as you want, any time you want. This is another case of "if it sounds too good to be true, it isn't." Many of these products are sweetened with such things as honey and molasses, which are as much of a problem to diabetics as table sugar. You also often get a lot of calories from the other carbohydrates and fat in the product. In addition, certain sweeteners such as sorbitol, mannitol, and HSH (hydrogenated starch hydrolysate) can have a laxative effect if they are eaten in excess. That's nature's way of keeping us from overdoing.

There are, of course, some calorie-free artificial sweeteners, such as Nutrasweet/Equal or saccharine. Although these are dietetically free for diabetics, because we don't yet know what's going to be revealed about them down the line we think it's best to follow diabetic dietitian Barbara Recio's "rule of two"—never have more than two servings of any one artificial sweetener in a day.

On the subject of artificial sweeteners, we've had repeated questions about the advisability of using an artificial sweetener during pregnancy.

Dr. Jovanovic: Artificial sweeteners have not been *proven* safe in pregnancy. It doesn't work the way the law does, where you're innocent until proven guilty. I consider artificial sweeteners guilty until proven innocent when it comes to their use during pregnancy. A word to the wise should be sufficient on this.

June and Barbara: For nonpregnant women who want to incorporate some sweeteners into their diet, Ron Brown has some advice on what they are and how to use them.

Fructose is a carbohydrate that has the same calories as sugar. But it doesn't raise the blood sugar as fast or as high, because it's processed and stored by the liver and delivered to the bloodstream as needed rather than just being immediately dumped into the bloodstream, the way table sugar is.

The catch is that you have to be under good diabetes control for fructose to have this advantage. If your blood sugar is high, then your liver gets confused, and fructose starts to shoot your blood sugar up as much as regular sugar.

Since fructose is a carbohydrate and has calories, you must limit its use. It's *not* a freebie. My suggestion is to use one-fourth the amount of sugar called for in a recipe as fructose and the other one-fourth as a saccharine-based noncaloric sweetener, such as Sugar Twin. You can usually leave out the remaining half of the sugar, since most desserts are too sweet anyway. The fructose helps cut the bitterness of too much saccharine, and the saccharine provides sweetness without adding extra calories or carbohydrate. If you're baking cake or cookies, though, sugar or fructose is needed for the structure, and generally you'd have to substitute the same amount of fructose for the table sugar.

Equal is the brand name of the very-low-calorie, noncarbohydrate sweetener Nutrasweet, which is the

brand name for the compound called aspartame. Nutrasweet has entered the sweetener arena in a big way. It's
in most diet soft drinks now and in several sugar-free
products. It's also in those little blue packets of Equal,
which can be used to sweeten anything from coffee to
chocolate mousse pie.

There's one major drawback to Nutrasweet, and that
is that you can't cook with it because it will lose its sweetness. Since Equal tastes better than the saccharine-based
sweeteners and, unlike fructose, has essentially no calories, it follows that it is the sweetener of choice for anything that doesn't have to be cooked. You *can* add it to
hot things such as coffee, but you just can't bake with it.

Ron mentioned fructose. We have found that fructose is used much more by diabetics in Britain and
Europe than in this country. In fact, *Balance,* the Journal
of the British Diabetic Association, recently published an
encomium to fructose, which we've reproduced in Appendix G. For *well-controlled, not-overweight* diabetics, fructose may be one way to have that occasional sweet treat.

Speaking of sweet treats, we've heard some research
that may help explain why so many women are "choco-
holics." (Incidentally, Ron considers this theory ridicu-
lous.)

But for what it's worth . . . some scientists have
discovered that eating chocolate produces the same
chemical in the brain (phenylethylamine) as falling in
love. That's why, when love has gone, people often go
on chocolate binges to try to recapture that certain feeling. To make a nonfeminist generalization, that may be
why there seem to be more women chocolate addicts
than men. Women tend to be more susceptible to love.
As Doris Lessing said, "Have you ever known a man who
would interrupt his career for a love affair—and have you
ever known a woman who wouldn't?"

But enough of sweetness and love, let's get back to the basics of nutrition in the diabetic diet.

On to another nutritional question. Diabetic women often ask us about taking vitamin and mineral supplements. We have the feeling that since a diabetic woman may have a limited diet, she may not naturally get enough of the vitamins and minerals she needs. What is your opinion about this?

Dr. Jovanovic: The recommended daily allowance (RDA) of calcium for a woman is 800–1000 mg, in order to prevent brittle bones in old age. As it turns out, diabetes, when it is out of control, tends to erode bones faster than in persons without problems of hyperglycemia. Therefore, it is best to stay in good diabetic control and to eat more calcium, just in case.

Growing girls and pregnant or lactating women need even more calcium—at least 1200–1400 mg per day in order to prevent a negative balance of calcium at these times of increased need.

All other vitamins and minerals tend to be in normal balance in persons with diabetes, no matter what the level of control. The following is a list of RDAs for all women, diabetic or not:

Vitamin A	800.0 mg
Vitamin D	5.0 mg
Vitamin E	8.0 mg
Vitamin C	60.0 mg
Thiamin	1.0 mg
Riboflavin	1.2 mg
Niacin	13.0 mg
Vitamin B_6	2.0 mg
Folate (Folic Acid)	400.0 mg
Vitamin B_{12}	3.0 mg

(Although B_{12} injections have been used as a treatment for diabetic nerve disease, there is no scientific proof that this works.)

Phosphorus	800.0 mg
Magnesium	300.0 mg
Iron	18.0 mg

(More iron may be needed if a woman has excessive periods or large blood losses with the delivery of her babies.)

A word of caution: Too much of a good thing may be poisonous. The vitamins and minerals that are toxic when taken in large doses include vitamin A, vitamin D, and iodine. Certain patients with iron-metabolism disease can get iron overload from too much iron. Thus, before embarking on a vitamin kick, it's best to consult a doctor about the right doses for you.

June and Barbara: There's more and more information these days on the importance of fiber in the diet, especially with those recent reports reaffirming that it helps lower cholesterol, prevent cancer of the colon, and discourage the development of diabetes. It's awfully hard to get enough fiber in the diet—especially when you eat out a lot. What, therefore, is your opinion of using a fiber supplement such as Fiber Excel to make sure you have enough? We have one Type II woman who reports (anecdotal evidence!) that she's lowered her blood pressure, weight, and blood sugar simply by adding the fiber supplement.

Barbara has started drinking a glass of Perrier with Fiber Excel in it morning and evening—especially when traveling. In Perrier it foams up and is like an oat soda. (It tastes a lot better than it sounds!) The reason she's something of a fanatic about it is that her father had a colostomy when she was in high school and she has hopes that fiber may win out over genes.

Dr. Jovanovic: Although high-fiber diets have been shown to decrease the prevalence of bowel cancer and to improve some forms of colitis, plus decrease the levels of cholesterol in the bloodstream when more than 50 percent of the diet is composed of fiber, there is still no scientific proof that a high-fiber diet is specifically important for a person with diabetes. Because fiber increases gas formation and thus can be a nuisance, I would wait for more studies of diet for persons with diabetes before prescribing high-fiber diets to all my diabetic patients.

June and Barbara: We know that the nutritional content of foods is vitally important. However, having written articles for such publications as *Gourmet, Bon Appétit,* and *Food and Wine,* we also feel that food is one of life's pleasurable experiences, not just a way of fueling the body or meeting the demands of insulin.

There's another important reason for having really delicious food. You need less of it to have a feeling of satisfaction. Consequently, it can help you control your weight. Dinah Shore, who at *un certain âge* looks lean and fit and terrific, does follow a good exercise program, but she also has a dining philosophy that helps. We once heard her say on a talk show that if she has, for example, a hamburger, she doesn't want it to be just a plain, average, run-of-the-mill hamburger that causes you to feel vaguely dissatisfied and hungry for more. No, she wants the *perfect* hamburger—a hamburger that makes you feel you've had a wonderful experience and that leaves you feeling comforted and full of good feelings.

You've probably noticed this yourself. When you have something absolutely delicious, you may seem to get filled up very fast. For that reason we always urge diabetics to become "food snobs." After all, food is, as has been said, the most intimate consumer product. You put it into your body and make it a part of your body, so you should want it to be nothing but the best. And, as a diabetic, since you must restrict how much you eat, you shouldn't stint on how good it is any more than you do on how good *for* you it is.

Take olive oil. We heard a radio report indicating that olive oil is the best oil to use to prevent heart disease. As evidence the report cited the fact that Italy and Greece—where olive oil is universally used—have the lowest rates of heart disease in the Western world. Olive oil, it was explained, is a monounsaturate. So is peanut oil, which they also recommended as a heart-disease preventer.

That was exciting news to us, because we love olive oil and use it more than any other kind in cooking. In fact, we consider ourselves minor connoisseurs of olive oil. But before getting all atwitter about it, we thought we'd better check it out with Ron, who said:

> Studies seem to show that saturated fats are the bad guys in elevating cholesterol levels and that both monounsaturates and polyunsaturates are the good guys. One group says that the polyunsaturates may be implicated in cancer, since they are more prone to oxidation. This is debatable.
>
> As far as cardiac risk goes, I would say monounsaturates are good in that they replace saturated fats, but they do not offer an advantage over polyunsaturated fats. Italians and Greeks don't use much butter or margarine, and they eat smaller amounts of meat. Therefore, their ratio of polyunsaturated and monounsaturated fat to saturated fat is quite high. That could account for the fact that they have fewer heart attacks.
>
> I personally like olive oil because it has lots of flavor, so you can use less of it than of the relatively flavorless

corn or cottonseed oils. Of course, for those watching their weight, using less *total* fat is important.

Peanut oil is good because it has a high smoke point, which means that you can get it very hot before adding food. In this way less oil is absorbed by the food.

Given this semiendorsement, we continue with our preference for olive oil. But, as we've suggested, it's best to get nothing but the best, or at least the second best. In case you want to follow in our olive-oiled footsteps, you should know that all olive oils are not created equal and that their labels can be rather confusing. *Extra virgin* (also called *double virgin*) is from the first pressing and is the most flavorful and expensive. *Virgin* is from the second pressing and is almost as good as the higher-priced oil. *Pure* olive oil comes from treating the previously pressed pulp with chemicals and is just adequate for cooking. *Fine* olive oil is like pure, except that water has been added. Use fine olive oil only in desperation!

Try these different oils, and you'll see how easy—and pleasurable—it is to become an olive-oil snob.

You can do the same thing with rice, experimenting with basmati rice in Indian dishes, arborio in Italian, and wild (which is not really a rice) in American and French. The more you learn about food and the more delicious food you eat, the less deprived you'll feel over the dietary restrictions of diabetes. Incidentally, your family and friends will likely be delighted to join you in following the diabetes diet, since this will be of great benefit to both their health and their taste buds.

Based on all our cooking and dining experience and our food snobbism, it's easy for us to be enthusiastic about following the diabetic diet. However, we realize to the uninitiated it probably doesn't sound like all that much fun.

Not long ago June was trying to cheer up a twelve-year-old girl who had just been diagnosed as having diabetes and, as is usually the case, had been stuffed full of diabetes information (translation: diabetes *restrictions*). June was telling her about all the possibilities for a cure, including the beta-cell transplants. The girl brightened up for the first time, and she asked, "When that happens, will I be able to eat anything I want?"

We realized again what a severe restriction not being able to eat anything you want is for most people. But it's 80 percent composed of a desire simply to *feel free* to eat anything you want. Feeling that you aren't free makes food you might normally shun seem infinitely desirable.

We were reminded of Mary Ellen Baran, who was one of the first persons to receive a pancreas transplant. After years of being a diabetic she suddenly *wasn't* one, and, boy, was she going to make up for lost time. We met her at breakfast during a diabetes conference. She was devouring pancakes that were swimming in maple syrup, and she told us that she had also been having a hot-fudge-sundae spree. She couldn't believe the miracle of being able to eat all the foods formerly forbidden to her.

We met her again a year later for lunch, and she was eating what appeared to be a perfect lunch for a diabetic. She had only a little fruit for dessert. What was going on? Had she turned diabetic again? Not at all. She told us that after a year of overindulgence in sweets and fats and anything else her formerly deprived heart and taste buds desired, she found that she had put on twenty pounds and felt perfectly rotten. She realized that this was no way to live, and she voluntarily went back to her former way of eating. In fact, she says she now follows a stricter regimen than she did as a diabetic, but she doesn't feel at all deprived because she's doing it by choice. As a result, she had slimmed back down and felt wonderful again.

So why don't you *pretend* that you've had a pancreatic transplant (who knows, you may have one before too long), and *pretend* that you've had your sweet-eating binge and gotten it out of your system, and *pretend* you're following your healthy eating plan because you want to look and feel good instead of just because you have to! You may just find that pretending—even more than wishing—will make it so.

ENVOI

NOT THE LAST WORD

What we've given you here definitely isn't the last word on the diabetic woman. There won't be a last word until the whole story of diabetes has a happy ending.

Diabetes is such a constantly changing field that even as as we write this, new discoveries are being made that could alter the entire picture. For that reason, we encourage you to keep asking questions, and we'll keep trying to give you the answers. Write to us at the Sugar-free Center, P.O. Box 114, Van Nuys, CA 91408. We'll forward your questions to Dr. Jovanovic and publish her answers in the *Health-O-Gram.* Even if you don't have any questions, write to us to get on the mailing list for the *Health-O-Gram* so you can learn from the questions other women ask. If we receive a tremendous influx of questions, we'll update the book or even write a new one.

Keep in touch. We're all in this together, and if we join forces, as Susan B. Anthony said, "Failure is impossible."

Appendix A

RECOMMENDED READING

Basic Books on Diabetes

Anderson, James W. *Diabetes: A Practical New Guide to Healthy Living.* New York: Arco, 1981.

Anderson cites many studies showing that fiber helps blood-sugar control. His diet—high in carbohydrate and fiber and low in fat (HCF)—can lower insulin requirements and eliminate the need for pills in Type II diabetics.

Belmonte, Mimi M. *Diabetic Child and Young Adult.* Quebec: Eden Press, 1983.

Belmonte of the Montreal Children's Hospital has been a specialist in childhood diabetes for over twenty-five years. This "primer for parents and professionals" is based on her conviction that it is possible and safe to normalize blood-sugar levels in children, and she tells you exactly how. Profound insights into all the life problems of young diabetics and their parents.

Bernstein, Richard K. *Diabetes: The Glucograf Method for Normalizing Blood Sugar.* Los Angeles: Jeremy P. Tarcher, 1983.

Bernstein, a Type I diabetic for forty years, is known as "the tartar of tight control." His scientific method requires six self-tests per day, multiple injections of insulin, and a high-protein diet. This pioneer book is of great value to Type I diabetics who are tired of their fluctuating blood-sugar levels and are ready to take charge of their diabetes in order to prevent complications and to feel their best twenty-four hours a day.

Biermann, June, and Toohey, Barbara. *The Diabetic's Book: All Your Questions Answered.* Los Angeles: Jeremy P. Tarcher, 1981.

Everything a newly diagnosed diabetic needs to know plus an updating for long-term and born-again diabetics. Special section for family members and friends.

Biermann, June, and Toohey, Barbara. *The Diabetic's Total Health Book.* New York: Pocket Books, 1980.

Focusing on your health rather than on your disease, this book provides you with the blueprints and tools necessary to build three impenetrable barriers to the effects of stress: a strong body, a tranquil mind, and a serene spirit. Tells how to choose and apply such effective therapies as progressive relaxation, autogenics, and visualization as well as use innovative techniques such as laughter and hug therapy.

Biermann, June, and Toohey, Barbara. *The Peripatetic Diabetic.* Los Angeles: Jeremy P. Tarcher, 1984.

Along with the original story of Biermann's diagnosis and how she faced diabetes on her terms is an update of her adventures seventeen years later. Tells how to overcome the despair of diabetes and learn to live a joyful and exciting life, full of dining, travel, skiing, and good times.

Ducat, Lee, and Cohen, Sherry Suib. *Diabetes: A New and Complete Guide to Healthier Living for Parents, Children and Young Adults Who Have Insulin-Dependent Diabetes.* New York: Harper & Row, 1983.

A coping manual for parents of diabetic children and for teenagers and young adults. Outstanding background on the emotional aspects of diabetes. Ducat is the mother of a diabetic and founder of the Juvenile Diabetes Association.

Lodewick, Peter A. *A Diabetic Doctor Looks at Diabetes, His and Yours.* New York: Bantam Books, 1987.

It takes a diabetic doctor like Lodewick to explain how things can go wrong even when you're doing everything right. Up-to-date information on all aspects of effective diabetes therapy. Special chapters for women, men, overweight people, and people over fifty. Never preachy and always optimistic.

Peterson, Charles, and Jovanovic, Lois. *The Diabetes Self-Care Method.* New York: Simon & Schuster, 1984.

A state-of-the-art manual that focuses on normalizing blood sugar through self-testing and insulin adjustment. The physicians who wrote this book, two of the country's foremost endocrinologists, believe that most complications of diabetes can be avoided, and they include a chart telling which ones are preventable and which are reversible.

Sims, Dorothea F., ed. *Diabetes: Reach for Health and Freedom.* St. Louis, MO: C. V. Mosby, 1984.

Dorothea Sims, editor of this self-care manual written by a team of health professionals, has devoted much of her life to working for diabetics and is herself an inspiring role model with forty years' experience as a diabetic. The book presents options rather than laying down rules. A large portion of it is devoted exclusively to the problems of Type II diabetics. Readable, compassionate, and supportive.

Diet and Cookbooks

American Diabetes Association and the American Dietetic Association. *Family Cookbook.* Vols. I and II. Englewood Cliffs, NJ: Prentice-Hall, 1980, 1984.

These two cookbooks are healthy eating guides for the entire family, not just the diabetic. Volume I includes 250 recipes, as well as information on nutrition, meal planning, exchanges, dining out, and fast food. Volume

II has 206 recipes, four chapters on fighting fat, an exercise program, ethnic dishes and exchanges, plus a section on fiber.

Bailey, Covert, and Bishop, Lea. *The Fit-or-Fat System Target Diet* and *The Fit-or-Fat System Target Recipes.* Boston: Houghton Mifflin, 1984, 1985.

These are the follow-up books for Bailey's fitness and weight-loss plan explained in *Fit or Fat?* The Target Diet is a clear, graphic way to help you avoid fats in your diet. The first book is an eating plan emphasizing losing body fat. The second is a recipe collection for delicious, low-fat dishes ideal for weight control for Type II diabetics.

Barrett, Andrea. *The Diabetic's Brand-Name Food Exchange Handbook.* Philadelphia: Running Press, 1984.

Calories and exchanges for 3000 foods from 400 manufacturers as well as ten fast-food menus. Vital for those with fast-lane eating habits.

Franz, Marion J. *Exchanges for All Occasions.* Minneapolis: International Diabetes Center, 1983.

This book contains 450 foods not found on the ADA Exchange Lists, as well as special lists for high-fiber, vegetarian, Chinese, Mexican, Jewish, and Italian diets and meals for camping, holidays, and lunch boxes. Essential for flexibility in dining.

Guilliard, Judy, and Kirkpatrick, Joy. *The Guiltless Gourmet.* Rancho Mirage: Nutrition Wise Partnership, 1983.

Written by a dietitian and a diabetic trained in classic French cuisine, this book contains sophisticated recipes from all over the world. All are computer analyzed for the diabetic diet, and all are low in fat, cholesterol, sugar, and calories.

Jones, Jeanne. *The Calculating Cook; More Calculated Cooking; Diet for a Happy Heart; Fabulous High Fiber Diet; Secrets of Saltfree Cooking.* San Francisco: 101 Productions, 1972, 1975, 1977, 1981, 1979.

Written by a nationally famous cook and diabetic who

specializes in superb food that's good for you, these four cookbooks make dining a joy. All recipes include exchanges.

Kahn, Ada P. *Diabetes Control and the Kosher Diet.* Skokie, IL: Wordscope Associates, 1984.

The only book that tells how to manage diabetes in accordance with Orthodox Jewish religious practices. In addition to three chapters of recipes there are low-fat and low-calorie adaptations of traditional Jewish dishes. Includes kosher exchange lists.

Kidushim-Allen, Deborah. *Light Desserts.* San Francisco: Harper & Row, 1981.

Many of the treats in this lovely book are more elaborate and satisfying than sugary desserts. Includes tips for cutting the fat, sugar, and calories in any dessert.

Loring, Gloria. *Kids, Food & Diabetes.* Chicago: Contemporary Books, 1986.

TV star Gloria Loring, whose son has diabetes, brings special understanding to family problems in this book of recipes, nutritional information, and coping skills. Gloria's personal help on these pages is like having a support group on your shelf at home.

Majors, Judith S. *Sugar Free Kid's Cookery; Sugar Free Microwavery; Sugar Free Sweets & Treats.* Milwaukie, OR: Apple Press, 1979, 1980, and New York: Ballantine Books, 1982.

These three books are approved by the Oregon Affiliate of the American Diabetes Association (ADA). *Kid's Cookery* recipes are easy for a young diabetic to prepare. *Microwavery* is a collection of 140 of Majors' speediest and tastiest creations. *Sweets and Treats* recipes are sweetened with fruit and fruit juices—no sugar or artificial sweeteners.

Marks, Betty, and Schechter, Lucille. *The International Menu Diabetic Cookbook.* Chicago: Contemporary Books, 1985.

With this book Marks, a diabetic, and Schechter make foreign cooking possible for diabetics. They present an amazing variety of exotic but easily prepared dishes that are not high in fat, including 300 recipes from eighteen countries and seventy-three menu suggestions. Includes exchanges, sources of foreign ingredients, and helpful hints.

Methven, Barbara. *Microwaving on a Diet; Microwaving Light and Healthy.* New York: Prentice-Hall, 1981, 1985.

Both of these books have mouth-watering illustrations and lip-smacking recipes. Both explain menu planning and include recipes from appetizers to desserts. Calories, sodium, cholesterol, and exchanges are given for each recipe. Everyone loves these books, not only for cooking but for armchair reading.

Middleton, Katharine, and Hess, Mary Abbott. *The Art of Cooking for the Diabetic.* Chicago: Contemporary Books, 1978.

A good first choice for a diabetic's cookbook library, this total food guide is by a diabetic diet counselor and a nutrition educator with diabetes in the family. It includes 300 recipes, low in sugar, saturated fat, and sodium.

Revell, Dorothy. *Oriental Cooking for the Diabetic.* Tokyo: Japan Publications, 1981.

Includes all of the old favorites of the Chinese and Japanese cuisines—egg flower and miso soups, egg foo yong, and tempura, lists calories and exchanges, and contains a special section on sodium-restricted recipes. Many recipes use the stir-fry method.

Robertson, Laurel, Flinders, Carol, and Ruppenthal, Brian. *The New Laurel's Kitchen.* Berkeley, CA: Ten Speed Press, 1986.

This book has everything for the diabetic who wants to be a vegetarian: 100 pages of sound nutritional information, inspiring philosophy, and recipes that open new vistas of dining happiness. The revised 1986 edition (updated from 1976) has 150 new recipes. Those from the first edition have been revised to lower their fat content and enhance their nutritional value.

Wedman, Betty. *American Diabetes Association Holiday Cookbook.* New York: Prentice-Hall, 1986.

Thanks to dietitian Wedman, diabetics no longer need feel deprived during the holiday season. Marvelous low-sugar, low-salt, low-fat recipes for traditional favorites like eggnog, fruitcake, latkes, and stollen. Also, many appealing, healthful dishes (pumpkin pancakes, barbecued prawns, broccoli soup) that can be enjoyed all year long. Includes vegetarian creations.

Exercise

Bailey, Covert. *Fit or Fat?* Boston: Houghton Mifflin, 1977.

For leading you into lifelong fitness, this book presents a twelve-minute-per-day aerobic exercise program that changes your metabolism, causing you to burn more calories even when you're sitting still or sleeping.

Biermann, June, and Toohey, Barbara. *The Diabetic's Sports and Exercise Book.* Philadelphia: Lippincott, 1977.

Exercise is not only the key to effective control of diabetes but the key to good health for everyone. And it has the added benefits of being free and fun. In this book over 150 diabetic sportspeople share their secrets and their experiences with you in every sport from lawn bowling to scuba diving.

Yanker, Gary. *The Complete Book of Exercisewalking.* Chicago: Contemporary Books, 1983.

How to design your own fitness program by converting walking into aerobic exercise and weight-control routines. Walking is an exercise almost anyone can do and enjoy. This book is full of information (on foot care, equipment, clothing, and supplies) and inspiration.

Pregnancy

Folkman, Jane, and Hollerorth, Hugo. *A Guide for Women with Diabetes Who Are Pregnant . . . or Plan to Be.* Boston: Joslin Diabetes Center, 1985.

Produced at the Pregnancy Clinic of the Joslin Center in Boston, this clearly written "labor of love" includes everything learned at the nation's first clinic to care for the distinctive needs of pregnant women with diabetes.

Franz, Marion, Cooper, Nancy, and Mullen, Lucy. *Gestational Diabetes: Guidelines for a Safe Pregnancy and a Healthy Baby.* Minneapolis, International Diabetes Center, 1985.

This booklet from the International Diabetes Center is for the woman who develops high blood sugars only during her pregnancy. The basic advice, however, is sound for all pregnant diabetics.

Stress Reduction

Biermann, June, and Toohey, Barbara. *The Diabetic's Total Health Book.* New York: Pocket Books, 1980.

This book's primary focus is on the role of stress in bringing on diabetes and in making its day-to-day control difficult to achieve. It explains what stress does, what the major stressors are, and how to overcome them. You can choose from an entire smorgasbord of innovative relaxation techniques, from autogenics to laughter and hug therapy.

Burns, David. *Feeling Good: The New Mood Therapy.* New York: Signet, 1980.

Psychiatrist Burns shows how, by changing the way

you think, you can alter your moods and get rid of low self-esteem, anger, depression, pessimism, and other "black holes" in your life, becoming rich in self-assurance and strength.

Glasser, William. *Take Effective Control of Your Life.* New York: Harper & Row, 1984.

Workable new ways to overcome problems and better control your emotions and your actions. Glasser's book shows you that misery is optional.

James, Muriel, and Savary, Louis. *New Self.* Reading, PA: Addison-Wesley, 1977.

Shows you how to make the positive changes in your emotional life that help you relate better to others and transform yourself into the living, loving, free person that you've always wanted to be.

Weight Loss

Bailey, Covert. *Fit or Fat?* Boston: Houghton Mifflin, 1978.

For helping you with weight loss or for leading you into lifelong fitness, this book describes how to change your metabolism by a twelve-minute-per-day aerobic exercise program. Use in combination with Bailey's *Fit-or-Fat System Target Diet* and *Fit-or-Fat System Target Recipes.*

Coyle, Neva, and Chapian, Marie. *Free to Be Thin; There's More to Being Thin Than Being Thin.* Minneapolis: Bethany House Publishers, 1984.

These two books rely on God and prayer for a successful weight-loss plan: "First Face God with the problem, then face the problem with God." They contain good advice for changing *any* behavior.

Franz, Marion, Hedding, Betsy, and Leitch, Gayle. *Opening the Door to Good Nutrition.* Minneapolis: International Diabetes Center, 1986.

Explains how to figure out what your weight should

be; how many calories a day to eat; how to plan your daily menus; and how to shop, cook, increase fiber, lower fat and cholesterol, and even determine what vitamins and minerals to take.

Katahn, Martin. *Beyond Diet: the 28-Day Metabolic Breakthrough Plan.* New York: W. W. Norton, 1984.

A twenty-eight-day program that causes you to lose weight at the rate of three pounds per week by increasing whole-body exercise such as walking, jogging, cycling, or rebounding. Good tips on low-calorie eating. Includes a pocket-size calorie and energy expenditure calculator. (Katahn's newest book, *The Rotation Diet,* is not recommended for diabetics.)

Appendix B

SUMMER CAMPS FOR DIABETIC CHILDREN

This list of summer camps for children and youth with diabetes is made available as a service of the American Diabetes Association. These camps are either sponsored or endorsed by their local ADA affiliate. If individual camps have financial-assistance programs available to help defray the cost of the camping session for qualifying campers, *Camperships available* will be written at the end of the entry. Check with the camp contact person for details.

Many ADA affiliates also offer additional camping programs such as day, family, and teen camps.

The Canadian Diabetes Association also offers camping programs; information about camps and day-care centers in Canada may be obtained from Canadian Diabetes Association, 78 Bond Street, Toronto, Ontario M5B 2J8. Telephone: (416) 362-4440.

The following camps are all accredited by the American Camping Association and have the designation "Y" (certified) as their program status.

Alabama

Camp: Camp Seale Harris
YMCA Camp Chanler
Rt. 7, Box 758
Wetumpka, Alabama 36092

Sponsor: American Diabetes Association
Alabama Affiliate, Inc.

Contact: Zula Walters, Camp Administrator
906 Coranada
Huntsville, Alabama 35802
Telephone: (205) 883-2556

Camperships available.

California

Camp: Camp Chinook
Camp Conrad (YMCA)
Angelus Oaks, California 92305

Sponsor: American Diabetes Association
Southern California Affiliate, Inc.

Contact: Sandra Benning
American Diabetes Association
Southern California Affiliate, Inc.
3460 Wilshire Boulevard, Suite 900
Los Angeles, California 90010
Telephone: (213) 381-3639

Camperships available.

Colorado

Camp: Camp Shady Brook
P.O. Box 1694
Colorado Springs, Colorado 80901

Sponsor: American Diabetes Association
Colorado Affiliate, Inc.

Contact: Arnold R. Schwanke, Executive Director
American Diabetes Association
Colorado Affiliate, Inc.
2450 South Downing Street

Denver, Colorado 80210
Telephone: (303) 778-7556

Camperships available.

Florida

Camp: Florida Camp for Children and
Youth with Diabetes, Inc.
Camp Montgomery
Montgomery Conference
Starke, Florida 32091

Sponsor: University of Florida
University of South Florida

Contact: Rhonda Rogers
P.O. Box 14136
Gainesville, Florida 32601
Telephone: (904) 392-4193

Camperships available.

Illinois

Camp: Camp Gran-Ada
Western 4-H Camp
R.R. 5
Jacksonville, Illinois 62065

Sponsor: American Diabetes Association
Downstate Illinois Affiliate, Inc.

Contact: Donna Scott, Executive Director
American Diabetes Association
Downstate Illinois Affiliate, Inc.
965 North Water Street

Decatur, Illinois 62523
Telephone: (217) 422-8228

Camperships available.

Camp: Triangle D Camp for Children with
Diabetes
Covenant Harbor Camp Site
Lake Geneva, Wisconsin

Sponsor: American Diabetes Association
Northern Illinois Affiliate, Inc.

Contact: Jean Harris, Camp Coordinator
American Diabetes Association
Northern Illinois Affiliate, Inc.
6 North Michigan Avenue
Chicago, Illinois 60602
Telephone: (312) 346-1805

Camperships available.

Indiana

Camp: Camp John Warvel
Happy Hollow
R.R. 2, Box 382
Nashville, Indiana 47448

Sponsor: American Diabetes Association
Indiana Affiliate, Inc.

Contact: Elaine McClane
Director of Programs
222 South Downey Avenue
Suite 320
Indianapolis, Indiana 46219
Telephone: (317) 352-9226

Camperships available.

Kansas

Camp: Camp Discovery
           Rock Springs 4-H Camp
           Box 55
           Junction City, Kansas 66441

Sponsor: American Diabetes Association
           Kansas Affiliate, Inc.

Contact: Carolyn Herl
           American Diabetes Association
           Kansas Affiliate, Inc.
           2312 East Central
           Wichita, Kansas 67214
           Telephone: (316) 265-6671
           1-800-362-1355 Intrastate

Camperships available.

Kentucky

Camp: Camp Hendon at Green Shores
           Green Shores
           Rough River Reservoir
           McDaniels, Kentucky 40152

Sponsor: American Diabetes Association
           Kentucky Affiliate, Inc.

Contact: Mary Ann Bowling
           American Diabetes Association
           Kentucky Affiliate, Inc.
           P.O. Box 345
           Frankfort, Kentucky 40602
           Telephone: (502) 223-2971

Camperships available.

Camp: Camp Korelitz
Camp Marydale
Erlanger, Kentucky
(See *Ohio*)

Louisiana

Camp: Camp Wawbansee
Rt. 2
Simsboro, Louisiana 71275

Sponsor: American Diabetes Association
Louisiana Affiliate, Inc.

Contact: Bob McVie, M.D.
Medical Director
P.O. Box 33932
Shreveport, Louisiana 71130
Telephone: (318) 674-6070

Camperships available.

Camp: Camp Whispering Pines
Independence, Louisiana 70443

Sponsor: American Diabetes Association
Louisiana Affiliate, Inc.

Contact: Jerome Ryan, M.D.
Medical Director
Medical Research Center
147 South Liberty
New Orleans, Louisiana 70112
Telephone: (504) 581-1574

Camperships available.

Maryland

Camp: Camp Glyndon
407 Central Avenue
Reistertown, Maryland 21136

Sponsor: American Diabetes Association
Maryland Affiliate, Inc.

Contact: Daniel Markowitz, Camp Director
American Diabetes Association
Maryland Affiliate, Inc.
3701 Old Court Road
Executive Park #20
Baltimore, Maryland 21208
Telephone: (301) 486-5515

Camperships available.

Massachusetts

Camp: Clara Barton Camp for
Diabetic Girls
68 Clara Barton Road
North Oxford, Massachusetts 01537

Sponsor: Clara Barton Camp Corp.

Contact: Shelley Yeager, Camp Administrator
68 Clara Barton Road
North Oxford, Massachusetts 01537
Telephone: (617) 987-2056

Camperships available.

Camp: Elliott P. Joslin Camp for Boys with
Diabetes
Richardson's Corner Road
Charlton, Massachusetts 01507

Sponsor: Joslin Diabetes Center, Inc.
Youth Division

Contact: Paul B. Madden, M.Ed.
Camp Administrator/Director
Joslin Clinic
One Joslin Place
Boston, Massachusetts 02215
Telephone: (617) 732-2455

Alternative Camping Program: One-week winter camp and weekend retreat programs for teenagers and families.

Camperships available.

Michigan

Camp: Camp Midicha
4205 Hollenbeck Road
Columbiaville, Michigan 48421

Sponsor: American Diabetes Association
Michigan Affiliate, Inc.

Contact: Lynn Crowe, Director of Youth Services
American Diabetes Association
Michigan Affiliate, Inc.
The Clausen Building, North Unit
23100 Providence Drive, Suite 475
Southfield, Michigan 48075
Telephone: (313) 552-0480

Camperships available.

Camp: Baycliff Health Camp (Midicha-Up)
Marquette, Michigan

Sponsor: American Diabetes Association
Michigan Affiliate, Inc.

Contact: Lynn Crowe, Director of Youth Services
American Diabetes Association
Michigan Affiliate, Inc.
The Clausen Building, North Unit
23100 Providence Drive, Suite 475
Southfield, Michigan 48075
Telephone: (313) 552-0480

Camperships available.

Minnesota

Camp: Camp Needlepoint
YMCA Camp St. Croix
Hudson, Wisconsin 54016

Sponsor: American Diabetes Association
Minnesota Affiliate, Inc.

Contact: Jean A. Acker, Director
Camping Programs
American Diabetes Association
Minnesota Affiliate, Inc.
3005 Ottawa Avenue South
Minneapolis, Minnesota 55416
Telephone: (614) 920-6796

Camperships available.

Mississippi

Camp: Camp Hopewell
Rt. 1
Oxford, Mississippi 38655
(See *Tennessee*)

Missouri

Camp: Camp E.D.I. (Exercise, Diet, Insulin)
YMCA of the Ozarks

Rt. 2, Trout Lodge
Potosi, Missouri 63664

Sponsor: American Diabetes Association
Greater St. Louis Affiliate, Inc.

Contact: Joseph T. Greco, Executive Director
American Diabetes Association
Greater St. Louis Affiliate, Inc.
1790 South Brentwood Boulevard
St. Louis, Missouri 63144
Telephone: (314) 968-3196

Camperships available.

Camp: Camp Hickory Hill
P.O. Box 1942
Columbia, Missouri 65205

Sponsor: Central Missouri Diabetic Children's
Camp, Inc.

Contact: Janet Held, Camp Director
P.O. Box 1942
Columbia, Missouri 65205
Telephone: (314) 443-2447

Camperships available.

New Jersey

Camp: Camp Nejeda
Saddleback Road
P.O. Box 156
Stillwater, New Jersey 07875

Sponsor: Camp Nejeda Foundation, Inc.

Contact: Janice Burd, Executive Director
Camp Nejeda
Saddleback Road

P.O. Box 156
Stillwater, New Jersey 07875
Telephone: (201) 383-2611

Camperships available.

New York

Camp: Camp Nyda
Burlington, New York 12722

Sponsor: American Diabetes Association
New York Diabetes Affiliate, Inc.

Contact: Albert Passy, Camp Director
American Diabetes Association
New York Diabetes Affiliate, Inc.
505 Eighth Avenue
21st Floor
New York, New York 10018
Telephone: (212) 947-9707

Camperships available.

Camp: Camp Hagoo
7 Hills Campground
Holland, New York

Sponsor: American Diabetes Association
New York State Affiliate, Inc.

Contact: Pat Knuezer, Director
Children's Hospital of Buffalo
219 Bryant Street
Buffalo, New York 14222
Telephone: (716) 878-7262/7000

Camperships available.

North Dakota

Camp: Camp Sioux
Turtle River State Park
Arvilla, North Dakota 58214

Sponsor: American Diabetes Association
North Dakota Affiliate, Inc.
and
Grand Forks Kiwanis

Contact: Mary Ann Keller, R.N., Executive Director
American Diabetes Association
North Dakota Affiliate, Inc.
P.O. Box 234
Grand Forks, North Dakota 58206-0234
Telephone: (701) 746-4427

Ohio

Camp: Camp Korelitz
c/o Camp Marydale
695 Donaldson Road
Erlanger, Kentucky 41018

Sponsor: American Diabetes Association
Ohio Affiliate, Inc.

Contact: Debi Price
4055 Executive Park Drive
Suite 100
Cincinnati, Ohio 45241
Telephone: (513) 733-8881

Camperships available.

Camp: Camp Ho Mita Koda
14040 Auburn Road
Newbury, Ohio 44065

Sponsor: Ho Mita Koda, Inc.
Diabetes Association of Greater
Cleveland

Contact: George Cervenka
Camp Director
14040 Auburn Road
Newbury, Ohio 44065
Telephone: (216) 546-5125

Camperships available.

Oregon

Camp: Gales Creek Camp
Star Route Box 1205
Glenwood, Oregon 97120

Sponsor: Diabetic Children's Camp Foundation

Contact: C. M. Emeis, Jr.
Diabetic Children's Camp Foundation
2519 North Mississippi
Portland, Oregon 97227
Telephone: (503) 282-0931

Camperships available.

Pennsylvania

Camp: Camp Firefly
Haim Road
Spring Mount, Pennsylvania 19478

Sponsor: American Diabetes Association
Greater Philadelphia Affiliate, Inc.

Contact: David A. Funck, Camp Manager
The Bourse Building
21 South Fifth Street
Suite 570

Philadelphia, Pennsylvania 19106
Telephone: (215) 627-7718

Camperships available.

Camp: Camp Setebaid
P.O. Box 475
Bloomsburg, Pennsylvania 17815

Sponsor: American Diabetes Association
Mid-Pennsylvania Affiliate, Inc.

Contact: Kathy Fries
ADA Field Office
P.O. Box 475
Bloomsburg, Pennsylvania 17815
Telephone: (717) 784-9133

Camperships available.

South Carolina

Camp: Did-Ja-Do-It
4-H Camp Bob Cooper
Lake Marion
Summerton, South Carolina 29148

Sponsor: American Diabetes Association
South Carolina Affiliate, Inc.

Contact: Earl W. Griffith, Executive Director
American Diabetes Association
South Carolina Affiliate, Inc.
P.O. Box 1699
Columbia, South Carolina 29202
Telephone: (803) 799-4246

Camperships available (in state).

Tennessee

Camp: Camp Hopewell
Rt. 1
Oxford, Mississippi 38655

Sponsor: American Diabetes Association
Tennessee Affiliate, Inc.

Contact: Doris Sears
American Diabetes Association
Tennessee Affiliate, Inc.
Tennessee Regional Office
80 North Tillman, Suite 109
Memphis, Tennessee 38111
Telephone: (615) 267-7129

Camperships available.

Camp: Tennessee Camp for
Diabetic Children, Inc.
2622 Lee Pike
Soddy, Tennessee 37379

Sponsor: Private, nonprofit

Contact: Mrs. Virginia Eddings
519 East 4th Street
Chattanooga, Tennessee 37403
Telephone: (615) 267-7129

Camperships available.

Utah

Camp: Camp Utada
Camp Roger

Sponsor: American Diabetes Association
Utah Affiliate, Inc.

Contact: Chuck Hand, Executive Director
American Diabetes Association
Utah Affiliate, Inc.
564 East 300 South
Salt Lake City, Utah 84102
Telephone: (801) 363-3024

Camperships available (in state).

Virginia

Camp: Camp Holiday Trails
P.O. Box 5806
Charlottesville, Virginia 22903

Sponsor: Private, nonprofit

Contact: Executive Director
P.O. Box 5806
Charlottesville, Virginia 22903
Telephone: (804) 977-3781

Camperships available.

Washington

Camp: Camp Orkila
Orcas Island, Washington 98245

Sponsor: YMCA and
American Diabetes Association
Washington Affiliate, Inc.

Contact: Carl Knirk, Program Director
American Diabetes Association
Washington Affiliate, Inc.
3201 Fremont Avenue North
Seattle, Washington 98103
Telephone: (206) 632-4576

Toll-free (Washington only):
1-800-628-8808

Camperships available.

Camp: Camp Sealth
         Vashon Island, Washington 98013

Sponsor: Seattle–King County Council of
         Camp Fire Girls and
         American Diabetes Association
         Washington Affiliate, Inc.

Contact: Carl Knirk, Program Director
         American Diabetes Association
         ·Washington Affiliate, Inc.
         3201 Fremont Avenue North
         Seattle, Washington 98103
         Telephone: (206) 632-4576
         Toll-free (Washington only):
         1-800-628-8808

Camperships available.

Wisconsin

Camp: Camp Needlepoint
         Hudson, Wisconsin 45016
         (see *Minnesota*)

Camp: Triangle D Camp for Children with
         Diabetes
         Lake Geneva, Wisconsin
         (see *Illinois*)

Camp: Camp Sidney Cohen
         Delafield, Wisconsin 53018

Sponsor: American Diabetes Association
Wisconsin Affiliate, Inc.

Contact: Sarah Batchelor, Program Coordinator
10721 West Capitol Drive
Milwaukee, Wisconsin 53222
Telephone: (414) 464-9395

Camperships available.

Wyoming

Camp: Camp Hope
Casper, Wyoming 82602

Sponsor: American Diabetes Association
Wyoming Affiliate, Inc.

Contact: Steven Johnson, Co-Director
Box 4568
Casper, Wyoming 82604
Telephone: (307) 265-5865

Camperships available.

The following camps are attempting accreditation and
have the designation "T" (attempting certification) as
their program status.

Arizona

Camp: Azda
Chauncey Ranch
Mayer, Arizona 86333

Sponsor: American Diabetes Association
Arizona Affiliate, Inc.

Contact: George F. Stoeberl, Executive Director
American Diabetes Association
Arizona Affiliate, Inc.
7337 North 19th Avenue
Phoenix, Arizona 85013
Telephone: (602) 995-1515

Camperships available.

California

Camp: Adanca Wilderness Camp (day camp)
Lafayette, California 94549

Sponsor: American Diabetes Association
Northern California Affiliate, Inc.
Alameda/Contra Costa Chapter

Contact: Shirley H. Jones, Chapter Coordinator
3100 Summit Street
5th Floor, South Building
Oakland, California 94609
Telephone: (415) 272-9155

Camperships available.

Georgia

Camp: Camp Liwidia
Camp Calvin (Session I)
Camp Rock Eagle (Session II)

Sponsor: American Diabetes Association
Georgia Affiliate, Inc.

Contact: Nancy Watkins
3783 Presidential Parkway
Suite 102

Atlanta, Georgia 30340
Telephone: (404) 454-8401

Camperships available.

Idaho

Camp: Camp Hodia/Hodia Wilderness Camp
Sawtooth National Forest

Sponsor: American Diabetes Association
Idaho Affiliate, Inc.

Contact: Don Scott
American Diabetes Association
Idaho Affiliate, Inc.
1528 Vista Avenue
Boise, Idaho 83705
Telephone: (208) 342-2774

Camperships available.

Iowa

Camp: Hertko Hollow
YMCA Camp
Box 182, Rt. 4
Boone, Iowa 50036

Sponsor: None

Contact: Vivian Murray, Camp Director
888 Tenth Street
Marion, Iowa 52302
Telephone: (319) 373-0530

Camperships available.

Louisiana

Camp: Lions Camp
P.O. Box 171
Leesville, Louisiana 71446

Sponsor: American Diabetes Association
Louisiana Affiliate, Inc. and
Louisiana Lions League

Contact: Johnette Frentz, M.D.
Medical Director
Tulane Medical Center
Tulane Avenue
New Orleans, Louisiana 70112
Telephone: (504) 588-5375

Missouri

Camp: Camp Shawnee
P.O. Box 22
Waldren, Missouri 64092

Sponsor: American Diabetes Association
Heart of America Affiliate, Inc. and
Camp Fire Girls

Contact: Mary Frances Arbeiter
Program Coordinator
9201 Ward Parkway, Suite 300
Kansas City, Missouri 64114
Telephone: (816) 361-3361

Montana

Camp: Camp Diamont
Hyalite Youth Camp
Bozeman, Montana

Sponsor: American Diabetes Association
             Montana Affiliate, Inc.

Contact: Mrs. Stanlee A. Dull, Executive Director
             American Diabetes Association
             Montana Affiliate, Inc.
             Box 2411
             Great Falls, Montana 59403
             Telephone: (406) 761-0908

Camperships available.

New Hampshire

Camp: Camp Carefree and Camp Pride

Sponsor: American Diabetes Association
             New Hampshire Affiliate, Inc.

Contact: Bev Hotaling
             Box 152
             Durham, New Hampshire 03824
             Telephone: (603) 868-2573

Camperships available.

New Mexico

Camp: Camp Triple D
             Camp Summerlife
             Box 22
             Vadito, New Mexico 87579

Sponsor: American Diabetes Association
             New Mexico Affiliate, Inc.

Contact: Mari L. Knopp, Executive Director
             American Diabetes Association
             New Mexico Affiliate, Inc.
             525 San Pedro, N.E.

Suite 101
Albuquerque, New Mexico 87108
Telephone: (505) 266-5716

Camperships available.

North Carolina

Camp: American Diabetes Association Youth Camp
Sertoma 4-H Camp
Rt. 1, Box 215
Westfield, North Carolina 27053

Sponsor: American Diabetes Association
North Carolina Affiliate, Inc.

Contact: Susie Piper, Camp Committee Chairman
4709 Charlottesville Road
Greensboro, North Carolina 27410
Telephone: (919) 294-5793

Camperships available.

Oklahoma

Camp: Camp O'Leary/Kno Keto
Camp Classen
Davis, Oklahoma 73030

Sponsor: American Diabetes Association
Oklahoma Affiliate, Inc.

Contact: Program Coordinator
American Diabetes Association
Oklahoma Affiliate, Inc.
6465 South Yale, Suite 423
Tulsa, Oklahoma 74136
Telephone: (918) 492-3839

Camperships available.

Pennsylvania

Camp: Camp Crestfield
R.D. #2, Box 71
Slippery Rock, Pennsylvania 16057

Sponsor: American Diabetes Association
Western Pennsylvania Affiliate, Inc.

Contact: Linda Siminerio, R.N., M.S.
Camp Chairperson
Western Pennsylvania Affiliate, Inc.
4617 Winthrop Street
Pittsburgh, Pennsylvania 15213
Telephone: (412) 647-2323
(412) 367-0357

South Dakota

Camp: Kiwanis Camp Haunz
Camp Rim Rock
Box 652
Rapid City, South Dakota 57709

Sponsor: Downtown Rapid City Kiwanis Club and
American Diabetes Association
South Dakota Affiliate, Inc.

Contact: Fennella K. Bergeson
Field Director
P.O. Box 659
Sioux Falls, South Dakota 57101
Telephone: (605) 335-7670

Camperships available.

Virginia

Camp: Camp William R. Jordan for Children with
Diabetes
Camp Makemie Woods
Barhamsville, Virginia 23011

Sponsor: West Central Richmond
Optimist Club and
Medical College of Virginia

Contact: Dr. Reuben B. Young
Box 65
MCV Station
Richmond, Virginia 23298
Telephone: (804) 786-0494

Camperships available.

West Virginia

Camp: Camp Kno-Koma
1036 Quarrier Street, #404
Charleston, West Virginia 25301

Sponsor: American Diabetes Association
West Virginia Affiliate, Inc.

Contact: Barbara Judy, R.N.
Camp Director
1036 Quarrier Street, #404
Charleston, West Virginia 25301
Telephone: (304) 346-6418
or
Toll-Free: 1-800-642-3055
(West Virginia only)

Camperships available.

Appendix C

DESIRABLE WEIGHT FOR HEIGHT (WOMEN)

Height	Small Frame	Medium Frame	Large Frame
4'10"	92–98	96–101	104–119
4'11"	94–101	98–110	106–122
5'	96–104	101–113	109–125
5'1"	99–107	104–116	112–128
5'2"	102–110	107–119	115–131
5'3"	105–113	110–122	118–134
5'4"	108–116	113–126	121–138
5'5"	111–119	116–130	125–142
5'6"	114–123	120–135	129–146
5'7"	118–127	124–139	133–150
5'8"	122–131	128–143	137–154
5'9"	126–135	132–147	141–158
5'10"	130–140	136–151	145–163
5'11"	134–144	140–155	149–168
6'	138–148	144–159	153–173

Appendix D

Activity	Calories Used per Hour
Strolling (1 mph)	150
Walking (2 mph)	200
Walking (4 mph)	350
Race walking	500
Jogging	600
Running	800–1000
Ballet exercises/ calisthenics	300
Cycling (5 mph)	250
Cycling (10 mph)	450
Tennis (doubles)	350–450
Tennis (singles)	400–500
Swimming (breaststroke or backstroke)	300–600
Aerobic dancing	600–800
Swimming (crawl)	700–900
Handball	650–800
Cross-country skiing	700–1000

Appendix E

DAILY CALORIE NEEDS

Age	Calories per day	Range
Birth to 6 months	Weight (lbs) × 53	43–66 (per pound)
6 months to 1 year	Weight (lbs) × 48	36–61 (per pound)

Children (Both Sexes)

1–3 years	1300	900–1800
4–6 years	1700	1300–2300
7–10	2400	1650–3300

Women

11–14	2200	1500–3000
15–18	2100	1200–3000
19–22	2100	1700–2500
23–50	2000	1600–2400
51–75	1800	1400–2200
Over 75	1600	1200–2000
Pregnant	normal + 300	
Lactating	normal + 500	

Adapted from recommendations made by the Food and Nutrition Board of the National Academy of Sciences–National Research Council, for average healthy people. Individual requirements vary according to weight, height, and activity level.

Appendix F

Appendix G

BRITISH DIABETIC ASSOCIATION
RECOMMENDATIONS FOR THE USE OF FRUCTOSE

Fruit Sugar—At Last, A Sugar for Diabetic Families
(Reprinted from BALANCE)*

If you're diabetic, or if there's a diabetic in your family, you've probably tried baking with most of the well-known sweeteners. And you've probably found that your cooking neither looks nor tastes as good as it does with sugar. So you'll be pleased to hear that there's now available a natural alternative that can be enjoyed in cooking by people with diabetes and their families. It's fruit sugar, otherwise known as fructose.

Just as ordinary sugar (sucrose) is the carbohydrate found in sugar cane, fruit sugar is an even sweeter carbohydrate found in sweet fruit and most vegetables. Fruit sugar does not contain any artificial ingredients, and has no bitter aftertaste that is commonly experienced with many alternative sweeteners. It tastes sweet just like sugar and has virtually the same calorie count (about 110 calories per ounce).

But there are two other very important differences. Firstly, it is sweeter than normal sugar, so not surprisingly you need less and hence consume less calories. And secondly, fruit sugar is absorbed much more slowly by your body and hence in small quantities does not give rise to severe highs and lows in your blood sugar level. What we're saying is that people with diabetes can use around 25 grams of fruit sugar in baking a day without jeopardising their control. That's the equivalent in sweetness to around 40 grams of table sugar. Or, to put it more simply, enough to bake a small sponge cake.

---

*Balance, June 1986, p. 30

On the subject of cakes, we should mention another property of fruit sugar. Tests have shown that using it in cooking actually helps to keep cakes fresher for longer. And in many instances, particularly with fresh fruit, it will noticeably enhance flavor, giving an overall taste that is better than with ordinary sugar.

The British Diabetic Association, who use fruit sugar in their baking recipes, also acknowledge that a cake mix made with fruit sugar needs much less beating than one made with an alternative sweetener, nor do you need to add extra fat to give it more bulk and to assist rising.

But if you're still at all sceptical, why not pick up a packet of fruit sugar and see for yourself? GUIDANCE FOR USE: Acceptable for use in baking and preserves. Remember to allow for the calorie content of the fruit sugar and, of course, the calorie and carbohydrate contribution from the other ingredients. FRUIT SUGAR IS NOT SUITABLE FOR THE OVERWEIGHT.

INDEX